Praise for *Seven Signs of Life*

"A brilliant, compelling account of what it is like to spend your days caring for patients 'on the fringe of existence' . . . A hugely life-affirming book. In between the many grim situations encountered on a daily basis, Abbey shows us moments of both joy and deep emotional connection."

—Kathryn Hughes, *Mail on Sunday*

"Heartfelt, honest, illuminating and wise—a wonderful book that I would urge everyone to read."

—Julia Samuel, author of *Grief Works*

"Illness is a thicket through which doctors and patients struggle—sometimes at odds, sometimes in concert. Into the harrowing penumbra between life and death come Dr. Abbey's signs of intelligent life. These seven cogent chapters probe the range of experience and emotions that patients, families, and medical workers must navigate. A welcome addition to the medical-literary canon."

—Danielle Ofri, MD, PhD, author of
What Patients Say, What Doctors Hear

"A powerful glimpse into the high stakes of intensive care. . . . Some readers may be wearying of doctor memoirs. This one . . . has a freshness and a sincerity that moved me. She is a gifted writer . . . honest, compassionate, sensitive . . . [and] the doctor we would crave in our greatest need."

—Melanie Reid, *The Times*

"A thoughtful and necessary book about a world all of us might inhabit at some point in our lives."

—Rosita Boland, *Irish Times*

"A wonderfully frank assessment of the emotions shared—and unshared—between doctors and their patients. . . . Dr Abbey writes movingly . . . and asks us all to think about what we want for ourselves at the end."

—*Daily Mail*

"Bold, courageous and most welcome. . . . Abbey imparts a wisdom concerning human emotional life that is sophisticated, and also simple and poignant. . . . If she is representative of an emerging generation of healthcare professionals, there is reason to be optimistic for the future of healthcare."

—Paul D'Alton, *Irish Times*

"A beautiful insight into the extraordinary highs and lows of intensive care. Dr Aoife Abbey writes with such sensitivity and obvious kindness about the emotions that define us all, doctors and patients alike. I was deeply moved by this wonderful book."

—Rachel Clarke, author of
Your Life in My Hands

"Effortlessly absorbing and illuminating . . . a prismatic set of arguments for a truth that we too often forget: doctors, nurses, and consultants are human, too . . . a perspective that feels like new territory. . . . Measured out in Abbey's crystalline, personable voice, it occurs to you that this is a somewhat Herculean feat."

—*Belfast Telegraph*

"A sensitive, honest, unsentimental and, yes, brave piece of writing that makes for compulsive reading."

—Nigella Lawson

"Aoife Abbey's honesty and insight are breath-taking. If you want to find out what it is really like to be a doctor, read this book."

—Dr Caroline Elton, author of
Also Human: The Inner Lives of Doctors

"Honest, compelling and compassionate . . . worthy of a place on the medical school curriculum. . . . This is a book with a warm heart, but also does not shy from honesty. . . . It's beautifully written, with valuable insights about how different patients and their families want different things from her and it is fascinating."

—Fergal Bowers, RTÉ

SEVEN SIGNS
of
LIFE

*Unforgettable Stories
from an
Intensive Care Doctor*

DR. AOIFE ABBEY

WITHDRAWN

ARCADE PUBLISHING • NEW YORK

Copyright © 2019 by Aoife Abbey

All rights reserved. No part of this book may be reproduced in any manner without the express written consent of the publisher, except in the case of brief excerpts in critical reviews or articles. All inquiries should be addressed to Arcade Publishing, 307 West 36th Street, 11th Floor, New York, NY 10018.

First North American Edition 2019

First published in Great Britain by Vintage. Vintage is part of the Penguin Random House group of companies.

Arcade Publishing books may be purchased in bulk at special discounts for sales promotion, corporate gifts, fund-raising, or educational purposes. Special editions can also be created to specifications. For details, contact the Special Sales Department, Arcade Publishing, 307 West 36th Street, 11th Floor, New York, NY 10018 or arcade@skyhorsepublishing.com.

Arcade Publishing® is a registered trademark of Skyhorse Publishing, Inc.®, a Delaware corporation.

Visit our website at www.arcadepub.com.

10 9 8 7 6 5 4 3 2 1

Library of Congress Cataloging-in-Publication Data is available on file.
Library of Congress Control Number: 2019943367

Jacket design by Erin Seaward-Hiatt
Jacket photograph © daboost/Getty Images (texture)

ISBN: 978-1-948924-82-5
Ebook ISBN: 978-1-948924-83-2

Printed in the United States of America

To my big brother Aaron, an activist. We miss you.
And to those who have trusted me, often without choice.

IX. The Four Ages of Man

He with body waged a fight,
But body won; it walks upright.
Then he struggled with the heart;
Innocence and peace depart.
Then he struggled with the mind;
His proud heart he left behind.
Now his wars on God begin;
At stroke of midnight God shall win.

W. B. Yeats, *Supernatural Songs*

Contents

Author's Note

THE EVENTS DESCRIBED IN this book are based on the author's own experiences and they have been collected over a period of years, from at least ten different hospitals or healthcare practice settings. While all of the events described are memories of real-world events, the names of patients, relatives, associates and colleagues, if used at all, have been deliberately changed. Additionally, personal and identifying details have been changed. This includes ages, genders, occupations, nationalities, appearances, familial relationships, medical histories and diagnoses. Any resemblances to persons living or dead that has occurred as a result of these changes will have occurred by coincidence.

Introduction

THERE ARE THOUSANDS OF doctors who, like me, spend their time walking in and out of a countless number of patients' lives. I have stood in rooms, stood in corners, sat on beds, sat on chairs and knelt on floors. I have been the visitor who was there when you found yourself most vulnerable, when you lay on a hospital bed or on a trolley in the emergency department. I have put my hands on you, and yet I have been somebody you may never even have known was there at all.

I am a specialist registrar in intensive care and I work on a national training programme for doctors who have finished medical school, worked through a further four years of postgraduate training and are now progressing towards the role of consultant intensivist. As a doctor in a training programme, I am constantly moving jobs and hospitals – so far, I have had eighteen separate jobs across seven years.

I don't think I have ever considered myself a writer, though I have always loved to read. I devoured other people's stories, but it was not until I had qualified as a doctor that I realised I might have some stories of my own. It is the human condition, I think, to try and make sense of things. There has never been a doctor who left medical school fully formed, and perhaps it was because I was so aware of all I had to learn that I started to write. Even seven years on from graduation, the more time I spend in intensive care, the more there is to make sense of. Seven years is a drop in the ocean.

It was more than two years ago that I took up the mantle as the British Medical Association's 'Secret Doctor' – an anonymous doctor whose task it was to write about 'everyday life' at work. 'The Secret Doctor' wasn't created to spy on people, whisper truths or blow any whistles. It was mostly created to start a conversation, as a way of suggesting to doctors that there were things we should perhaps talk about more. The intention was to bring together doctors at all points of their career, and the anonymity incumbent in that role was always about focusing the conversation not on the writer, but on the topic at hand. The vision was less about creating a celebrity doctor and more about building a community that could celebrate and discuss, with appropriate honesty, what it is to be a doctor. At least that was the sort of role I had in mind.

Fulfilling this remit meant being honest: about what I knew, and what I didn't. It meant inviting opinions on my own experiences and problems, and it meant writing in a way that lent itself to readers, not just from a healthcare-profession background, but from the public, too. It meant wanting other people to join in.

It also involved thinking a lot about how I felt.

When I took the time to stop and really scrutinise how my job made me feel, I realised the incredible scope of things that I had simply got used to. I realised how strange all the things I had been conditioned to take in my stride might seem to someone who has never walked in my shoes.

I am not talking solely about the advancement of medicine and technology, though I am surrounded daily by the complex equipment we have created in a bid to scupper illness and disease. Instead I am talking about the large part of my job that is reliant not on being able to work with instruments, numbers, drugs and machines, but on being able to work with being human.

Of course ongoing academic achievement and the acquisition of hard skills are paramount to a doctor's development, but they are not the whole story. Many of the pivotal moments in any doctor's story are about learning how to talk to people, to understand them and to make yourself understood. Competence is not simply about knowing what is possible, but also about understanding what is right. It is about feeling and, more importantly, about knowing what to do with a feeling.

Within the context of what I do in intensive care, you will see that many of my patients are often not just vulnerable, but also temporarily dwelling in another place: sedated and mechanically ventilated. I look after people who are at the extreme fringes of existence, and intensive care can be a realm rendered both inaccessible and strange. When I speak to patients or their families and I feel that a conversation hasn't gone well, sometimes it seems this is because of the power imbalance that my job creates. There can be a sense that I know, or have access to, an understanding about things that give me the upper hand.

I often think relatives might feel the sting in this because I am the one with the apparent knowledge – the passport to this world that has taken possession of their loved one. Yet they are the ones who feel it is their job above all to advocate the life of that person they have come to support. They are the ones who are often stuck: frightened, angry, grieving; feeling as if they are waiting to lose everything, or something close to it. It doesn't seem fair that we cannot, at the very least, set off on an equal footing.

The particular point that I want to share with you about the field of medicine I am training in is this: that for all the expensive equipment, all the technology, the screens, the drugs, the lines and the numbers, much of what my world is centred around are feelings that you are already deeply familiar with.

In biology class, you might have learned about 'the seven characteristics of living things'. These are the signs that tell you that a mouse is alive, but that a stone on the beach is not. All of the things that we call 'living' share, at the most basic level, this collection of traits: movement, respiration, sensitivity to their surroundings, growth, reproduction, processes of excretion and the utilisation of nutrition.

I think I always knew that the particular organisms I wanted to spend my life working with were humans; and between humans there is another sort of commonality that is shared. It is the experience of the emotions that hold us all together: fear, grief, joy, distraction, anger, disgust and hope. Yes, they often exist within the context of my own day, as emotions on some form of anabolic steroid. They are often pumped up, oversized and bulging. Across one shift, I might be privy to the spectrum of highs and lows that another person might hope to encounter only over a lifetime. But these feelings are still versions of exactly what you already know. When one doctor stands at the head of a trolley looking down at a patient who is dying, surviving or still somewhere in between, you would be forgiven for focusing on everything that sets those two people apart in that moment. All of the differences between them are obvious. But isn't it more likely that we are all exactly the same? What my time as a doctor has taught me so far is that all of the things I most need to come to terms with are the very same things I have been dealing with since the day I was born: those signs of being human.

Let me show you what I mean.

Fear

I learned that courage was not the absence of fear, but the triumph over it ... The brave man is not he who does not feel afraid, but he who conquers that fear.

Nelson Mandela

I WANT TO TELL you that I am brave. I want to tell you that the doctor standing at the head of the bed, while you take up the role of 'possibly dying patient' on a trolley, is courageous. I hope that I am, but it has become convenient for me to forget that would not be true, but for the acknowledgement of fear.

The first time I felt fear at work it was almost comedic in its ridiculousness, and it took me by surprise. If someone had taken me aside in medical school and asked me what I thought I might be most afraid of at the beginning of my career, dead people wouldn't even have made the list. The thing is, I come from a background where death and dying aren't taboo. In my family, we 'wake' our relatives in their homes, and the coffin is usually open. The first body I ever saw was when my grandmother died. She was laid out in her best clothes on top of her own duvet on her own bed. I remember being eleven years old and sitting on the bed beside my cousin, chatting about things unrelated to death or funerals, whilst absent-mindedly rearranging the rosary beads around her cold, dead fingers.

My first job as a doctor was on an elderly care ward and, for obvious reasons, it didn't take long until the issue of a dead patient presented itself. I don't think I had even considered it might be my job to 'verify' death, until the first opportunity arose (you will have to forgive this use of the word 'opportunity' – as a doctor, opportunities to learn often occur in the setting of unfavourable events). I found myself approaching the registrar to tell him that I had no idea how I was supposed to go about it. He took me to the patient's bedside and we went through the steps together. When the next time came round, though, I was on my own. I entered the side-room alone and shut the door behind me. I put on gloves, which in retrospect seems odd, because I wouldn't have put on gloves to do a routine external examination the day before, when the patient was alive, but now they were dead, and I was already acting differently.

I approached the bedside and I remember being especially put off by my realisation that this patient was still quite warm. When I placed my stethoscope on her chest, I could hear those hollow noises that rumble inside the thorax of somebody who is dead – the sort of noises that make a newly qualified doctor think: What if they're not dead at all? What if I say they are dead, and then the family walk in the door and she moves? These are the sort of noises that make you wish you'd waited until the patient was colder.

Verification of death involves looking in the pupils, checking for a response to pain and stating that there is no respiratory effort, no palpable pulse and no heart sounds. The last three take some time, so I stood for the requisite two minutes with my stethoscope on her chest and my hand on her neck, where you would find a carotid pulse in a living person. And I stared. The more I stared at that patient, the more I became convinced that she was going to open her eyes. I pictured them snapping open, her hand lurching towards where I had my hands on her neck, and her grip closing itself around my wrist, clamping shut with a strength that I knew she did not have in recent life. I let my imagination construct the whole terrifying ordeal; I couldn't stop it, and when the second-hand signalled the passing of two minutes, I raced out of the room, heart pounding.

It reminds me of something I used to do in my first childhood home. We had a staircase that went straight upwards – the house was built in the Seventies, and the first seven or so steps had empty spaces between the treads. As a child, I would convince myself that a hand was about to spring from one of those holes and grab me round my ankles. It wasn't real, I knew it wasn't, but I let myself believe it and I ran so fast up those stairs. Perhaps it is true that we create most of the fear we experience.

Looking back on this first experience of verifying a death, I still remain surprised by how I felt. Why hadn't I felt this way around a dead body previously? Maybe it was the corpse of somebody whom I did not already love that made the difference. Perhaps it was because it was *my* job to say they were dead (and what if they weren't?).

I don't know if I've ever experienced undiluted fear quite like that again, though I do think that at least some of what I do requires a level of courage. And how can I call myself brave, if I cannot admit to still feeling fear?

One afternoon as a still-green, first-year registrar in intensive care I was waiting in the emergency department for a middle-aged man who'd had a myocardial infarction. We had been alerted in advance and, on that particular day, heart attacks were like buses: there had been no emergencies for hours and then, just as the evening shift started, two arrived at once. We split our teams accordingly and things got busy.

Martin was wheeled in, red-faced and drenched in sweat. His appearance was typical of somebody in cardiogenic shock. This is what happens when the heart suddenly becomes unable to do its job, which under normal circumstances is a task of two halves: the

Aoife Abbey

heart receives deoxygenated blood into its right side and sends that blood to the lungs to be oxygenated, before receiving it back into its left side and pumping it out into the body again. In the medical sense, 'shock' can refer to a number of sudden insults to the body, all of which leave a person unable to supply their tissues and organs with sufficient circulation to support them. In Martin's case, the culprit was what is called a myocardial infarction or 'heart attack', and disruption to the blood flow through his coronary arteries meant that his heart muscle was dying a little bit more, with every second that passed us by. 'Time is muscle,' the cardiologists like to say. And so when Martin arrived, it was with the remit that there was no time to lose.

A quick glance told me that he was somewhere between conscious and not. He had the noisy, snoring hallmark of a partially obstructed airway and he was obese, with a body mass index that was at the very least fifty. Even on a good day, Martin wasn't made for lying flat and it was clear he would require induction of anaesthesia and the insertion of an endotracheal tube to protect his airway. So this will be my first solo emergency intubation in the emergency department, I thought as

I looked at him, and exhaled slowly. I find I am rarely presented with the 'average 70-kg man' that they write about in textbooks.

The cardiology consultant was lingering at the bedside, eager to speed up Martin's passage into the catheter lab, and he had already summoned the rest of the on-call intervention team. 'We need to get moving,' he told me. 'Are you happy with his airway?'

Of course I wasn't happy with his airway. Martin was far too unwell to support his own breathing while lying flat on a table in the coronary catheter lab. I prepped for intubation: drugs, laryngoscope, endotracheal tube; mental walk-through plan A, plan B, plan C. One of my more senior colleagues was in the bay next to me, preparing for the other incoming patient, and there was a pre-hospital emergency-medicine consultant another cubicle away. I took this in and reassured myself that I would have help, if I ran into trouble.

I looked down at my patient as he lay on the trolley. He was huge, clammy and snoring. But he *was* snoring – breathing for himself. I looked at the syringe of muscle-paralysing drug in my hand and thought how I would soon put a stop to that. About forty-five seconds after

the drug entered his circulation, he would stop breathing and then, for some seconds, his life would hover
precariously in the space between here and the 'there'
that I hoped I would keep him from.

Airway, Breathing, Circulation: we like to make the
routines of emergency care accessible to the memory in
a crisis. So we have a pre-formed plan of attack: airway
first, breathing second, circulation third. I have been
drilled on these manoeuvres and it can be as easy as
ABC, but if I couldn't manage the A and the B, Martin
would be dead in minutes. Even if I managed the A and
the B flawlessly, if I didn't judge the drugs correctly,
I might bring about the end of his already-failing C.

If you had come up to me at this point and asked,
'Are you afraid?', I'd have told you No and that, clinic-
ally, I was competent to be in this position. It was my
job. I'd have said I had a plan and a healthy amount of
respectful apprehension, but I was not afraid. Bowing
to fear is something that happens when you're not in
control. What help would that be to me?

I was afraid.

As I was making some final adjustments to the
trolley, trying to angle Martin's head so that it did

not extend so far backwards, in contrast to the tower-ing height of his abdomen and thorax, I looked up and saw an emergency-department consultant whom I hadn't seen in at least two years. He remembered my name. 'How are you?' he asked. It seemed at the time an odd moment to start bedside chit-chat, but I know now that wasn't his motivation for approaching me.

I told him of my plan for Martin's airway, my 'plan A' and my back-ups, and then he asked me if I'd like him to be on his merry way or to stand quietly in the corner behind my left shoulder. I chose the latter. We pulled the curtains around our bay and I sent Martin off to sleep. I waited the seconds that seemed like hours for paralysis to set in and for him to stop breathing. During this time my grip was vice-like beneath his mandible, as I pulled up the angle of his jaw to keep his airway open, while keeping the oxygen mask pressed onto his face. We waited and my eyes flicked back and forth from his gradually slowing chest to the monitor beside me, until there were no more breaths and forty-five seconds had passed. Before I start an emergency intubation, I always say the same thing to the nominated nurse or doctor on the team: 'If his oxygen saturations drop below ninety per cent, tell me. If I don't answer you, I didn't hear you, so tell me again.'

I picked up the laryngoscope, guided it into Martin's mouth and proceeded to pull the weight of him up, and then up with more force. There, exactly where they were supposed to be, were the vocal cords: gateway to the trachea, pathway to the lungs. It was a perfect view. I pushed the tube through the hole, inflated the cuff, hooked him up to the portable ventilator and it was done. Martin was prepped for the catheter lab, ready to have his coronary artery unblocked.

The consultant had only made two comments during the entire procedure, and he said them quietly enough that only I could hear him: 'This is going really well' and 'You're doing great.'

In that moment I needed to believe in myself, and not succumb to the fear that was threatening to rise up at any second. Looking back now, it's clear from the consultant's kind words that it was blindingly obvious to him this was what I needed. As doctors, I think we often choose to make fear cryptic, by calling it something else: apprehension, trepidation, acknowledgement that something is serious, nervousness, lack of confidence.

Any of these feelings we might freely admit to, but 'fear' is not a word that we often use. Frequently I am involved in the resuscitation of a patient and the only outward signal that I am frightened is the bead or two of sweat that starts to drip slowly down the small of my back. There are times when I peel off my gloves and am genuinely surprised by just how wet my palms have become. There are times when I fool myself.

I extubated Martin myself during a night shift, a couple of days later. He'd had a rocky few days, but he did well subsequently and went back to his life; to his wife and their two Labrador dogs, which he now intended to walk every day. When a patient is 'ready' to have the tube out, they are often more than ready. The plastic becomes an unwelcome irritation within their throat, and their eyes water with the discomfort because, unsedated, they fight against its presence. I lean towards Martin, so that my face is in his eyeline, and say, 'Don't worry, we are going to get this tube out now.' His wide eyes implore me to, and in that moment I am aware that he has placed a palpable amount of trust in me. I am also aware of the privilege. I remember pulling the tube out, hearing his now-hoarse, thick West

Country accent and thinking how nice it sounded. It is a strange thing to have been through something that was, for different reasons, so significant to both of us, and yet to share no real relationship at all. I'd never even heard Martin's voice until that moment.

There have been occasions when I was even less sure-footed in the face of fear. George Eliot said that 'we learn words by rote, but not their meaning; that must be paid for with our life-blood, and printed in the subtle fibres of our nerves'. From the first day that I started working as a doctor, I knew what a 'Do not attempt cardiopulmonary resuscitation' (DNACPR) order was. I knew what it meant; I knew the indications for it and I knew the implications of it. But more than three years into my career, I stood with a patient and a DNACPR order, and fear made me question everything I knew.

It was 4 a.m. and I had found myself on the way to the oncology ward to see a woman in her fifties. Her nurse was worried about new-onset shortness of breath and a fast heart rate, so she had paged me and done an ECG (electrocardiogram). I was on-call at that time for medicine, providing urgent reviews and troubleshooting whatever problems cropped up during the night. As was the usual way for out-of-hours cover, the vast majority of those patients weren't part of my daytime caseload; I didn't 'know' them.

I reached the ward and was met by a woman sitting on the edge of her bed. She was about the same age as my own mother and was very short of breath. I estimated a respiratory rate of more than thirty breaths a minute. Her oxygen saturations were less than 90 per cent, and I still recall thinking how seemingly calm and composed she was, for somebody who was struggling so obviously. The nurse went to get another oxygen mask and I enquired if the woman had any pain.

She shook her head and replied, 'No pain.' Her tone carried no urgency; it was as if I'd asked her if she had wanted sugar in her tea.

'Are you sure?' I reiterated. 'You don't have *any* pain in your chest?'

'No,' she said. 'I just came back from the toilet and felt breathless.'

'And can you slow your breathing down?'

'I don't think so.'

The nurse returned with the new oxygen mask, as I placed my stethoscope on the patient's back and listened to her breath sounds; air moved in and out of her lung fields, and they sounded clear. Much too clear.

'I'll be back,' I said, as I left her behind me to look at the ECG, which had been placed on the nurses' station outside. The pattern of right heart strain was obvious and confirmed my suspicions: this woman had a massive pulmonary embolus.* I had never diagnosed an immediately life-threatening pulmonary embolus myself, and I'd never seen one before it had been treated. Nevertheless, I felt sure of it. I picked up her folder of notes and there, poking out of the front cover, was the DNACPR order. It had been discussed and signed just two days before, citing reference to discussion with the patient, and metastatic cancer. I remembered only in that instant that I was on the oncology ward.

---

* A pulmonary embolus occurs when a blood clot exists in one of the pulmonary blood vessels. In the case of a massive pulmonary embolus, the blood clot blocks one or both pulmonary arteries. In doing so, it puts the right side of the heart – whose job it is to receive deoxygenated blood from the body and pump it into the lungs to be oxygenated – under great strain.

So here I had a woman who I was sure had a massive pulmonary embolus, who was probably about to have a cardiac arrest, but hadn't done so yet, and the form for limitation of treatment only mandated that we wouldn't carry on after that happened. There was no other advice, but I knew she would never be given thrombolysis to break down the clot – the risk of bleeding from her tumour would be astronomical – and yet I was not sure if I could make that decision, alone in the middle of the night, as a relatively junior doctor, for a patient I hardly knew. I had picked up the phone to call the medical registrar when the nurse called from the patient's bedside, 'You better come back in here, Doctor.'

My patient now lay flat on top of her bed: breathing, heart beating, but unresponsive. Seconds ticked past and I was helpless, standing there thinking that I owed her something, but I did not know what. She had walked to the toilet, and now she was dying so abruptly that this nurse at the bedside and I were the only two people who knew about it. Who else was supposed to know? The nurse said she would go and call her family, although I realised the patient would probably be dead before they arrived. I couldn't bring myself just to leave this woman alone while I went to call the medical registrar.

When you read this story, you may pause time for a while, to consider what you might do next. But, in that moment, time surrounded me like an army advancing: step, step, the sound of heavy boots on ground, rifles brandished with their bayonets pointed in. Time, breathing down my neck; so close to me that I could hardly think. No time to think at all. I asked the nurse to put out a medical emergency call, too.

Within minutes the team had assembled: registrar, intensive-care junior, another medical junior and two night sisters. I gave them a short summary, and the medical registrar uttered the short response that I knew he would: 'She isn't for CPR.'

'Yes, I know,' I defended myself half-heartedly, 'but her heart is still beating and I just ...'

I just what? I just didn't know if it was okay for me to stand and watch this death? I just didn't feel at home here? Whose mother was this? I wanted to say, 'There wasn't time to call you personally and I didn't know what to do.' I just felt there was no time. I just felt afraid.

Before I had explained myself, the night sister interrupted and said, 'You did the right thing.' I was more than grateful for those words. Within seconds, I felt my patient's pulse slip away from her wrist beneath the grip of my hand on hers, and then she was dead. At 4 a.m., at the end of a third-floor corridor, on a ward that I did not know, with a patient I had only just met, in a situation I felt could not be salvaged, I needed to know that I was making the right decision and I needed to know that I wasn't alone.

When I first wrote a version of this experience for a blog piece, an anonymous doctor posted a comment underneath. It said: *'the fact that the night sister said you did the right thing did not make it the right thing to do ... you are emotionally needy ... [she] put a period to your sentence to save you from being berated'*. Part of the doctor's point was correct, of course – I had called a medical emergency team to a patient who was imminently, and unavoidably, dying. I had called them for support, both clinical and emotional, but I don't apologise for either. Telling somebody they 'did the right thing' is a subjective accolade. Would it have been right for this doctor, who felt so strongly that I was doing the wrong thing, to call the medical emergency team and ask for help? Perhaps not, if he or she was more experienced than me, and perhaps he or she would have been more sure of themselves. But was it right for me in that moment? For a doctor who was inexperienced and had never diagnosed a massive pulmonary embolus? For a doctor who was scared, faced with high stakes and worried there was even a minuscule chance that there was something else that could be done, beyond standing there and watching her die? Yes, it was the right thing for me; and yes, I would know better next time.

But was it the right thing for my patient? I don't believe it was, entirely. The best thing would have been for me to sit calmly, hold her hand and be present with her for her death. That wasn't the doctor she got that night; I did not have that presence of mind, and I don't mind admitting it.

The medical emergency team had left again within minutes, but the night sister and I waited on the ward together to tell her family what had happened. Though I have been involved in so many such situations now, there are individual parts of these conversations that remain indelible. What I most recall about this one was that her husband asked me if she had suffered, at her end. I told him no, that I thought she had fallen away from any sort of knowing quickly, and that she was gone in the blink of an eye.

I've said that doctors have coping strategies to explain away fear. Mostly this happens unconsciously – the goal is to micromanage it in that moment, because it does not do for both doctor and patient to succumb to fear. You cannot be a rabbit in the headlights – it simply isn't helpful. As an intensive-care doctor, it is the nature of my work that my patients are often afraid. In many ways, their fear becomes routine. It is something I expect, and there is a standard reassuring phrase that I have come to say, in the first instance: 'Don't worry, everything is going to be okay. We're all here to keep you safe.'

This doesn't mean that I think every patient's fear is the same. When I call a patient's fear 'routine', it is not a value judgement, it is just part of *my* routine. The sort of work I do often doesn't leave a lot of time to work conscientiously through the origins of fear with a patient. They need something, urgently, and you are required to deliver it, urgently, whether or not they're frightened. So you find yourself focusing on reassurance, and on the emergency words that come to mind while you are trying to deal with the emergency: everything is going to be okay, we've got you. Though I've often wondered if it really is all right to say that. Frequently I don't actually 'know' if it will be okay at all. Frequently, nobody does.

But in practical terms, what else can you say? Mostly I anaesthetise or send people 'off to sleep' when they are *in extremis*: when they are struggling to breathe, when they are struggling to stay alive. It is not unusual for me to be in a situation where the patient is more than likely going to die either way; but trying to prevent it is appropriate, because there is actually a chance you can help. It is what the patient has asked you for, and it remains the best hope they have.

There is a lot about today's society that looks unfavourably on doctors who venture to question if the paternalistic 'doctors know best' attitude might still have a place in modern medicine. For the most part, I agree with them entirely, but there is a limit to how honest you can realistically be, in the seconds you might have to talk to the critically unwell patient in front of you.

I'm not sure why on this occasion specifically, but one day I tried an approach that was less paternalistic in its reassurance. The patient had been thrown through a windscreen in a car accident. He was a young male in his twenties, well built, with tattoos on his arms and a chain around his neck. He was bleeding, a lot, and I had found myself in the position of keeping my hand pressed on his previously gushing neck-wound. Understand-ably, my hand was pressed down firmly. He complained that I was hurting him and asked me to 'get the fuck off' him. I told him, nicely, that I couldn't move my hand because I was trying my best to keep him from bleeding.

'Am I going to die?' he asked suddenly.

'We're doing absolutely everything we can to help you. I know it is hard, but I need you to try and stay calm, so we can sort you out and get you to theatre.'

Louder: 'But am I going to die?'

'You've got some significant wounds; we're going to get you to theatre and do everything we can to make sure that doesn't happen.'

Now shouting: 'AM I GOING TO DIE?'

He wanted a definitive: a yes or no, and I could have chosen either, but they would both have been a lie. I had no guarantees.

At this point the resuscitation practitioner jumped in with: 'No, you are not going to die!' He then gave me a look that said, 'What's got into you?' The patient went quiet immediately, and we got back to doing what he needed us to do, in the full knowledge that, in fact, yes, he might die.

Outside the remit of controlled situations, giving reassurance is often what you have to do, and I think the people who would judge me harshly for this aren't the ones actually bleeding out or struggling to breathe on the trolley. The reality is that some patients look at you through their terrified, dilated pupils and they want you to say it's going to be okay. In the end, either I am right and they will be okay, or I am wrong and I will live with the fact that I chose to tell them otherwise.

'Don't worry, everything is going to be okay. We're all here to keep you safe.'

I was working for the anaesthetic department and the consultant and I were anaesthetising Peter, a patient in his late sixties, for surgery. Peter had come in with a large abscess that required incision and drainage. It was unplanned surgery, in the broad sense, but in contrast to what I do now, there was no real extra life-threatening risk, outside what you would normally associate with a general anaesthetic. Peter was visibly nervous, so I smiled reassuringly and tried to make my eyes look as kind as possible. I pressed the plastic oxygen mask gently onto his face and told him to relax and breathe normally, while the consultant drew up the drugs and checked that the cannula in the back of Peter's hand was working. I stood behind him and wondered what my own face must look like, as he saw it, upside down.

Peter was fidgety and kept telling me he just wanted 'this all to be over with'. I told him it would all be over before he knew it.

Patients in hospital exhibit different amounts of fear. One patient might crumble at the sight of a needle, and yet the next patient might not bat an eyelid; and most patients behave somewhere in between. Apart from screaming children, I really don't think I've seen a more nervous patient than Peter in the anaesthetic room. But as a doctor, you learn to expect the full spectrum of behaviours, and an excess of fear just becomes something else that you do your best to manage.

'Is it normal to be frightened?' Peter asked.

I answered him that yes, of course it is; and I remember reminding him that having surgery isn't something that happens every day – if he didn't feel worried about it, that wouldn't be normal.

Truthfully, I didn't judge his fear. Losing control of your life, even for an hour, is a frightening prospect. I've only had a general anaesthetic once; it was when I had all four of my wisdom teeth out, and I was already at medical school then. In the moments I spent waiting in the anaesthetic room I found myself wondering what it might feel like to be on death row, about to have a lethal injection. I thought about what it might feel like to be remorseful and yet still have no control over the fact that I was about to die. I really got into it, and the last thing I remember saying as I drifted off to sleep was a panicked plea: 'No, I've changed my mind, I don't want this any more.'

When Peter had spent about three minutes breathing in the oxygen from that mask I held over his mouth and nose, we continued the process of induction. The consultant picked up the collection of syringes, ready to start the anaesthetic.

First drug. Second drug. Watching the patient. Watching the monitors.

'This doesn't feel right,' Peter muttered drowsily as he drifted down into the sleep we had induced.

'Don't worry,' I replied calmly, 'everything is ...' and before I reached the end of my sentence, he was unconscious. I touched his eyelashes with my index finger, gently, to observe the absence of any reaction.

Third drug. Eyes on the patient. Eyes on the monitor.

Flush the cannula. All is okay. Wait. I looked at the consultant, who nodded to me to lift the laryngoscope and then, finding the view, I inserted the endotracheal tube without difficulty. I glanced at the monitor and removed the laryngoscope, resting it on the pillow next to Peter's head. In the brief seconds it took me to do that and look again at the monitor, he had, without any sort of ceremony or warning, had a cardiac arrest.

We started CPR immediately. We did all the things you do to try and drag a life back into a room. Our team got bigger and bigger, and we went through every step there was to go through, but four hours later, Peter was still dead.

There are lots of things I remember about that day. I recall being grateful that we had taken a proper pre-anaesthetic history and that we hadn't cut any corners. I remember the experience of seeing the consultant, standing in the aftermath. There was absolutely no fault involved, but I recall the devastation on his face, and his colleague telling him to go home and let her take over the rest of his work that day. I remember trying to sleep that night and allowing myself to wonder what Peter had wanted to eat when he came round from his surgery, and what plans he had for the summer. I recall wondering which of his family members would miss him the most.

I also remember wondering if I was strong enough to cope with the burden of telling patients they would be all right, when actually there was always some chance – however remote – that they might be dead. I recall asking myself if maybe it wasn't my job to take away a patient's fear, and maybe I didn't want that responsibility anyway. Usually what was happening to them was bloody frightening; often they had a decent chance of dying, and usually when I said they were going to be okay, as if I somehow knew that for a fact, I was, technically, lying.

But you go to work the next day and stare into the next set of terrified eyes. That patient's fear explodes into the moment that you share together, so how can you not respond by taking their hand and telling them everything will be all right?

Just over a year after qualification, there was a patient whom I looked after on the neurosurgery ward. Lara and I were about the same age, and she was one of those patients that doctors refer to as 'fit and well', until she had a seizure at her office, and then another and another. She worked in payroll, but talked about studying at night to be a counsellor. I'd been looking after Lara for almost two weeks while she waited for various investigations, a brain biopsy and a diagnosis. Normally I'd enjoy going to visit her, but on this particular day I ended up avoiding her, because I knew she was getting a visit from the oncology team, and I knew her brain tumour was of the worst possible kind. I really hadn't started off the day planning to avoid her, but earlier Lara had asked me if I was all right and she'd mentioned that she thought I was acting differently. I feigned tiredness, changed the conversation and then kept myself away from her, until the proper team had a chance to break the news.

Later that afternoon I walked into her room. She was sitting on the side of her bed with her feet on the floor. She looked up, met my eyes and said, 'I presume you know?'

'Yes,' I replied. 'I'm sorry.'

I shut the door behind me and sat down beside Lara on the edge of the bed, and we both looked straight ahead. I don't often sit side-by-side with a patient like this, like old friends on a park bench, except that, instead of watching the world pass us by, we were staring at the sink on the wall opposite us. And I was dressed in smart clothes for work, while Lara was dressed in pyjamas.

'Well, I'll be okay, won't I? I get the impression this won't shorten my life?'

Lara's question took me by surprise. It wasn't surprising that she had asked it, but I think I was surprised that she had asked me. She looked frightened, like I'd never seen her look before, and as if she wanted to ask the question, but possibly hadn't decided if she wanted to know the answer.

In my head I recalled that the five-year survival rate for this type of brain cancer was about 6 per cent. How could she ever have drawn the conclusion 'this won't shorten my life' from a conversation about her tumour? Why had she not asked the oncology team? For some reason she had chosen to ask me instead, and now I was sitting in a room with her; with her fear and mine.

The fear panicked me and I paused. I wasn't the expert, and actually how well did I know Lara at all? Well enough to know if she wanted the whole truth, or simply a version of it? Well enough to know what was in her best interests?

She must have read something in my expression, as she repeated her question, adding, 'If I'm wrong, I'd rather know now, while it's just me here.'

I took a breath; I explained to her that I was not an oncologist, but I knew that she had a high-grade tumour, and that part wasn't good news. I told her there were positive things about her individual case: she was young, without other chronic illness; she had already had a resection of her tumour and now had a clear plan for ongoing treatment. I watched Lara's face carefully, but she didn't stop me, so I continued: there were also things that I did not know. I didn't know if the tumour margins had all been removed successfully; I could not tell if it would grow back; and I did not know how she would respond to the treatment.

'But in the end, yes, there is a very real chance that this is going to shorten your life.'

'Yes' had never seemed like such an enormous word.

There were a few quiet seconds. My eyes glanced down at the white skirting boards and up again towards the sink on the wall, and then Lara said, 'Thank you for telling me.' I turned to look at her and she gave a half-smile, of the sort I can only describe as revealing expected disappointment. It wasn't resignation, but perhaps acceptance that, in asking the question, she had taken a step towards seizing control of what she needed to know. I didn't add further to that explanation, but I sat with her for a while longer and we spoke about how upset she felt that she would bring so much worry and grief to her family. I reminded her that she could not stop her family from loving her, and it was their prerogative to do so. I said that it was early days, and that I hoped in time she would be able to free herself from the burden of feeling responsible for their pain.

Had I been truthful? I had not lied, but I had not been as explicit as I could have been. I had not given her the five-year survival rate that she would find on the Internet. I wanted to tell Lara the whole truth, but when I spoke, those other words were captured by the enormity of her question and by the fear that comes from knowing that what is said cannot be unsaid.

Lara died within two years. I am sure that she had multiple more frank and expert discussions with her oncologists and palliative-care team after that. It is possible that she did not, after a time, even remember those minutes in a room with me, but I often think about that conversation and, when I do, I wonder whose fear was more palpable: hers or mine?

I think patients under the pressure of unexpected illness are often not the person they would recognise as themselves. The world around them can become unfamiliar and at that time, when they are so vulnerable and exposed, they are reliant on strangers – people who, if they had passed them in the street the day before, they would not have even said hello to. As a doctor in these moments, I think I inevitably become somebody who doesn't entirely belong to me; somebody I perhaps wouldn't easily recognise. I become somebody defined by the enormity of what that patient needs.

I once went to see a man on the ward after he'd been discharged from intensive care. Earlier that month he had been in a road-traffic accident; he'd broken multiple ribs, his arm, part of his pelvis and his collarbone. He'd also had some nasty lung contusions and required a tracheostomy and a prolonged period on a ventilator. Now he'd had his tracheostomy removed and was well enough to move to the ward. I was passing by, so I popped in. We were chatting about how good it was to be in a room with a window once again and some natural light, when he stopped abruptly and declared, 'Aren't you small?'

'What do you mean?' I asked.

'I don't know, I hadn't realised how tiny you are, love.'

He was no longer critically unwell, no longer so dependent on what I had to offer him. I was the same doctor, but having left the critically ill part of his journey behind him, he felt taller perhaps; and now I was noticeably just 5 feet 2½ inches tall.

I have distracted frightened children with YouTube videos and teddy bears, so that somebody can put a cannula into their hand. I have stood by an MRI machine with a claustrophobic patient while she had her whole spine scanned and have massaged her feet, because it helped her get through the scan, which she needed in order to plan urgent radiotherapy to shrink the cancer that had deposited in her spine. I have promised local anaesthetic to the patient who is terrified of needles.

Sometimes, though, patients hand you their fear and you can do absolutely nothing about it. There is no control; no question to be answered; no trick, no procedure to be done. That is the sort of encounter that really clings to my bones.

'I am just so frightened – everything has changed so quickly.' These were the words of ninety-three-year-old Michael. Despite the fact that macular degeneration had left him able to see only shapes and shadows, Michael still lived independently, and his mind was sharp. Unfortunately he had recently fallen at home. And, in an instant, the wheels had stopped moving; he had come to hospital and we had shown him that he was old. Hospital is often lamented as no place for the old; it is so often not a friend to those who fight to remain fit.

The physiotherapy team came to see him, but Michael now had pain in his joints. Over the time he'd been recovering from the fall, his bones had got used to the bed-rest and so we gave him a pain patch. He sat at the end of a six-bedded bay. His poor eyesight meant that he could no longer read, and the patient next to him was in no fit state for conversation. The other doctors, nurses and I did our best to engage him. We chatted about current affairs, and I found myself phoning various dead-end leads to source him some audiobooks – anything to stop his mind going on holiday, too. I found myself defending Michael in referrals. There was a roll of the eyes from some colleagues when his age slipped from my lips and it set my defensive barriers soaring up, like walls. I wanted to shout, 'Don't write my patient off!' I wanted to ask them if they knew that Michael had managed a farm for his entire life. I wanted to ask them if they knew that he had wanted to be a painter; or that his teacher had slapped him for writing with his left hand. I wanted them to know that he had told me who he was planning to vote for in the next elections.

'I am just so frightened – everything has changed so quickly.' His words had imprinted themselves inside my head: he had laid his fear at my feet, and how could I not fight to keep him safe from it? But there was also a rhyme that played ominously in the background: 'All the King's horses, and all the King's men, couldn't put Michael together again.'

Michael never went back to his own home – he stayed with us for a few weeks and regained some of his mobility, before moving on to a care home. He seemed calmer; he was glad to leave hospital and happy that there would be a garden at the new care home. Not long before he left the hospital, another junior doctor and I took Michael outside in his wheelchair. The day had been quiet for us, it was sunny and one of the beauties of an old district general hospital is that they often offer outside space. Michael asked us to describe the flowers. His son arrived for a visit and we all sat in the garden, facing the sun.

After some minutes Michael turned to me and asked, 'Can you explain to my son about what we said the other day – you know, about that resuscitation?'

We had had a conversation a few days beforehand, Michael in his chair and me on his bed, and I'd asked if he had ever thought about what he might want at the end of his life. What did he want to happen when his heart stopped? It took courage for me to approach Michael that day. His fears were still raw in my ears, and yet I was about to confront him with something intrinsically linked to his own mortality. We discussed CPR and the limitations of this 'treatment'. When we had finished the main thrust of our discussion, he stopped to think for a moment or two and then asked me if I thought God would mind if he just accepted death. I told him I wasn't an expert on God, but I didn't think He would.

So now, sitting in the garden, I began to explain to Michael's son the basis of his decision not to accept CPR at the time of his death. Then we went back to talking about the weather and how nice it was to feel the sun on our faces.

When I consider the faces of fear that I encounter, it can be ones with less urgency that weigh most heavily.

Fear

Michael's fear of becoming less able, in the context of his advancing age, was heartbreaking, and the impetus to reframe that fear was almost overwhelming. There is a human reflex, I think, to want to hand fear back to people as something else, and to reshape it. I could have smiled and said, 'Don't worry, you are going to be back on your feet before you know it', but without the excuse of immediately life-threatening urgency, it did not seem like the right thing to do. You try to allow a patient's fear to be present, even if you risk feeling their pain yourself.

I met Gloria when I was less than a month qualified. She was ninety years old and had been in hospital for many weeks. She was frail and had become immobile with pneumonia. She spent her last weeks in a side-room on the elderly care ward. Even with two hearing aids, Gloria couldn't hear very well; you had to shout at her to make yourself understood. If, like me, your accent wasn't local, you had to shout – and shout slowly.

We reached the point in Gloria's care when it was clear that she was in the last days of her life. I remember

45

standing by her bed one morning, when she gripped my hand suddenly and, looking at me with desperation, said, 'Please, don't let me die.'

What could I do? You can't say, 'Of course you are dying, Gloria; you are ninety years old, you have been dying for weeks and I can't change that now.'

I tried to explain, to soothe her, but she couldn't hear me through her anguish, and it's not the sort of conversation that lends itself to shouting at someone. As a new doctor, I don't think I expected elderly people to be frightened of dying. I guess it is just easier if they are not; easier for me, anyway.

I would prescribe Gloria the correct medications to help her death pass as comfortably and painlessly as possible, but that didn't seem helpful enough, and I felt in that moment more powerless than I had ever expected to feel. I found the registrar and told him what had happened, but he brushed me aside; maybe he felt helpless, too.

I couldn't shake it off, so I called the consultant. I told him that I thought Gloria needed emotional support and asked whether it was okay to ask her family if they knew she felt this way? Was it all right to put that on *them*? I didn't want to be cruel to Gloria's family, I told him, but I had just left her begging me not to let her die, and I didn't know what to do. This was the first consultant I had ever worked for, and although I liked him for many reasons, looking back, it was the comfort of knowing he would always take my worries seriously that made him so valuable to me, as a first-year doctor. That day I don't know what I would have done if he hadn't given me his time.

The consultant suggested we should phone and invite the family in that afternoon for a conversation. With apprehension, I asked them if they had any thoughts about how Gloria was feeling. As it turned out, they had already suspected she was frightened. It was already on their minds, and they thought what would bring Gloria comfort was a chaplain. It seemed like such a straightforward and obvious answer. Why did I not think of it myself? Confronted by her fear, I had panicked because I had no medical solutions.

Two of our hospital chaplains came, and they each spent some hours with Gloria. Each time I walked past her room and glanced through the window, I saw her lying in her bed with a chaplain seated nearby, their hands folded on their lap in that peaceful way they do. Gloria died that night, sooner than any of us had expected. I believe the chaplains gave her what she needed – that which I couldn't give her – and I don't think she died frightened.

I like to think that Gloria's fear became something else. If you are lucky, I believe that is what happens. Your fear of death becomes an impetus to find comfort. Your fear of losing your hard-fought independence becomes the momentum you need in order to stand on your feet again. Your fear of becoming the reason your family must experience grief gives you the strength to seek out truths that it may be painful to hear.

And the fear of standing over a patient, with their life in your hands, becomes the push you need to work to a standard where you can always look back and know that you did your best.

Grief

Perfect devices: doctors, ghosts and crows. We can do things other characters can't, like eat sorrow, un-birth secrets and have theatrical battles with language and God.

Max Porter, *Grief is the Thing with Feathers*

I CANNOT PUT A number on the times I have stood amongst the grief of families, or at least a part of it. I am aware that what I see is really just an opener for what is to come: the tip of an iceberg looming on the horizon of a family's life. I have a small part in the opening act, but it is their show.

At medical school I learned about grief in a classroom. They tell you that grief is mostly normal; but it can become pathological. And they tell you that it is your responsibility to break bad news well. If I am honest, little of what I learned in medical school actually prepared me for my role in these situations, but there are some things that you just have to commit to learning as you go along.

It is now almost seven years since I graduated as a doctor and, when it comes to breaking news, there are three rules I have picked up so far:

1 Listen.

2 Always say the words 'dead', 'death' and 'dying' (if that is what you mean).

3 Never, ever promise anybody anything that isn't yours to promise.

Perhaps that doesn't seem like a lot of wisdom to show for seven years of practice, but the truth is that, aside from these constants, I simply try to do my best. A doctor walks into a room and how can they ever really know for sure what is going on inside the head of the relative in front of them? It is of course better for everyone if we strive to believe that we *can* break bad news well; taming that beast is a noble pursuit, but it is vanity to forget that grief is not always a predictable thing. Grief has so many faces.

Sometimes grief will just walk out of a room: walk, run, storm or march.

One morning I was one of three humans in a room with magnolia walls, green plastic armchairs, framed flowers in watercolour and an unbranded box of tissues on the table between us. I said, 'Hello, my name is ...', introduced the nurse beside me and then explained what it was that I did here in intensive care. I asked the daughter opposite me what she understood about what had happened so far to her mother. I listened and filled in some gaps in the story, before progressing to the main event.

I was the human with the news – the bad news; the chief in charge of the breaking.

As medical students, we are taught formally about the concept of imparting bad news 'successfully'. I have been to lectures, sat through role-play with actors, reflected on films and on real events. Developing the skills required to break bad news has always been high on my list of priorities, but I often wonder if any of us really know what this means. When I remember that particular day in that magnolia room, I tell myself that I could have done it better. I recall that I *have* done it better, many times. That was not, after all, the first pin that I had pulled from a grenade, and it was not the first one I had thrown. You might imagine – despite the paucity of information I have given you – that you could have done it better. You might be right.

On days like that one, when I am left with the feeling that things haven't gone as well as I am conditioned to believe they could have, I always come back to the same question: well means well for whom, anyway? Who was I actually trying to keep sane, in that room? *I* might feel better if I did not have to sit in the wake of a slamming door, or pore over the words that I had used, but that other human's mother was about to be plucked from her life and who was I, really, to try and conquer her gut-wrenching reaction to that truth? Who is anyone to say that she was ever even mine to control? That death, that grief – neither existed at my bidding.

I told this girl of not yet twenty that her parent was dying today, that she will never wake up and know life as we think she would have liked to know it. I told her that truth, and then I told her something softer, something that might be considered more beautiful; something about comfort and care and peace.

Grief

But on that day, grief shifted in the green plastic armchair. Grief closed its eyes, shook its head and refused to take receipt of what I had presented. I gave her silence and then told her I was sorry for her situation, and that I could only imagine the hurt she must feel. Grief answered that she was not hurt; she was annoyed. She had every reason to be annoyed.

So she stood up and said, 'No, that is enough.' She lurched for the doorway and, in her panic to leave the room, her hand fumbled and slipped from the handle of the door. She grabbed it again, this time successfully securing her desperate exit from the scene, and I did not stop her. The door slammed behind her. The nurse, or I, would follow her; but not yet.

After conversations like this one, I am supposed always to ask myself: How could I have done that better? How could I have thrown a grenade into that person's life and *not* compelled them out of the chair and out of the room? But sometimes I honestly think that there have to be situations where the other person was always going to run out of the room. Sometimes I think that part of the trick to breaking bad news well might be having the strength to accept that you *are* actually breaking something.

At medical school, they try to make the teaching 'real'; the actors I was faced with in role-play were enthusiastic, sometimes to the point of irritation, and I might have scowled and accused them of enjoying the role of 'confused and grieving relative' a little bit too much. None of that really prepares you for quite how intrusive and raw the grief of another person can feel.

It was 9 a.m. and I had just helped a nurse pick a woman up off the floor of intensive care. She had rushed to the hospital and then fainted on being confronted by her moribund brother; short-circuited and collapsed under the weight of it. She wilted down to the floor and we put a pillow under her head. When she had rebooted and slowly opened her eyes, I watched a gradual realisation creep over her face that nothing had changed, before the pain frosted back over her eyes. Her brother, aged barely thirty, was intubated and ventilated and perhaps an hour away from circulatory death, when his heart would stop. This family had been gathered by a consultant that morning and told his imminent death was now inevitable. For all intents and purpose, he was dead enough for a family to start to grieve. In intensive care, grief often needs to start before a heart stops.

Minutes later, I was standing in a side-room with the same family and their dying relative. There were two sisters now, a brother, and the brother who would soon leave them. My team had felt that a side-room would offer the family more privacy in their grief, and I had just helped to transfer my patient there from the main ward. I was finishing up and gathering some items to take out of the room, when the shouting began. They started shouting at their brother, demanding that he come back. One of his sisters grasped his shoulders and shook him, and perhaps her grip did not raise his shoulders up from the bed that harshly, but I remember how violent an act it seemed, when contrasted with the inanimate slumber-state of the patient, his eyes closed and his body covered only by a white sheet.

Then his brother turned to me and, shouting now, his voice cracking in despair, said, 'Come on! You have the machines – we just want you to try!' They looked alike, these brothers, although one had a face that lay placid and unknowing, while the other face looked on, contorted and now increasingly agitated. This face turned back to me and shouted louder, 'Why aren't you trying? Do you want money?'

Nobody waited for me to answer, before one of the sisters took over and tried a different approach; she asked me if I knew how important he was to them, if I knew how much they all meant to each other? I told her that yes, I could imagine. I told her that I also had a brother and that I was really sorry for their situation. I tried to sound somehow kind, calm and caring, but I also said no, there really was nothing I could do to change the outcome. The family tore around the room, not knowing what to do with themselves or the situation, and then, when their frustration tired, they sank silently into chairs or onto the floor.

There was so much sadness in that room, so much desperation, but for all the anguish and pain that filled the space, I don't think I will ever understand what *I* actually felt. I think what I felt was emptiness.

A family is in pain, and it just isn't about you. Empathy is often exalted as the undisputed key value of modern medicine and patient-centred care. Feelings of empathy are laden with opportunity for personal bias, and there are, after all, some occasions when actually experiencing the tragedy and pain of a patient or family in front of you is largely superfluous, or even detrimental to the job you need to do. I don't think anyone has ever told me that it can be okay sometimes, or even useful, to build a wall between the pain in front of you and your own psyche. But I think it is. There have been plenty of times in my career when I have favoured a more limited version of compassion over actual empathy; and there have even been times when deliberate detachment from some of a family's words was what I needed to do.

I have been called a murderer. On that occasion it was the early hours of the morning and I found myself standing with a family who had that night been told that their relative had sustained sudden unsurvivable brain damage. This woman had been driving down the motorway one moment, and had pulled over with a headache the next. Between these two things, an aneurysm inside her head had burst. Driving. Dying. One seemingly mundane event had transitioned silently into something catastrophic. An ambulance hurtled down the motorway towards her, and there was nothing silent about the aftermath.

I had been part of the receiving team; I had cleaned the vomit from her soiled airway, pushed the tube into her trachea, squeezed the bag to inflate her lungs and struggled to overcome the extent of aspiration of stomach contents, which had made its way down into her smaller airways. I went down her tube and into her lungs, with a camera called a bronchoscope; sucked and washed that mess until we could at least establish enough oxygenation to keep her alive. By the time she was stable enough to take through a CT scanner, where the catastrophic extent of her haemorrhage was confirmed, she was already as good as dead.

The consultant had come earlier and explained the hopelessness of the situation. I now stood with my patient and her family after we had transferred her to intensive care, and they still had questions. It is normal to need to hear things more than once, so I reiterated to her family that she could not survive now, with or without our ventilator to help her breathe, or our drugs to try and keep her heart and blood pressure stable. Then I elaborated that there was no surgical option, nothing that time could do; and as I handed out these truths, the patient's husband towered over me and then said, in a matter-of-fact way: 'If you take the tube out of her, you will be a murderer.' He was talking about the tracheal tube that allowed us to ventilate her mechanically.

I raised my eyes to his and absorbed his words. In that situation you explain, with all the slow consideration and compassion that is required, that death is not just an option – it is an inevitability. On that particular day I explained that their relative could not live now, and that I could not save them. I explained that even if we left her intubated and on a ventilator, this woman's heart would still stop today, or perhaps tomorrow. I told them that their loved one would never wake up and live again, that I was sorry and that I understood this must be devastating news for them to hear.

Without blinking, her husband looked at me again and said, 'Yes, I know, but I am telling you that is how *I* will see it. *We* will see it like that; you *will* be the murderer.'

As a doctor in this kind of situation, you don't get to behave as if somebody on the street has accused you of something terrible. You don't get to behave as though you've been accused of wanting to commit an unspeakable act. There is no room for justified consternation or impassioned cries of denial, because this isn't about *you*. Say it inside your head, it helps: *This is not your show*. You are there firstly to be what your patient needs you to be, and secondly to be what the people whom that patient loved need you to be. So yes, I will stand and listen to a family tell me that if we accept the inevitability of death, so that this patient might have a death that we feel is more dignified, the family will look back and see me not as the person who received their loved one into the resus department, and who worked as part of the team that did everything in their capability to keep them alive, but as the person who killed them.

Then I wait and, when they need me to be something else, I am that, too.

That patient died the same day. I returned for my next night shift around the time that her heart came to a stop. She died, still ventilated and on full health support; I presume it was important to them that she did. I told the family how sorry I was for their loss, and no one made any reference to their previous accusations. The husband said thank you, and his brother met my gaze, wordlessly. Then they exited from intensive care, with their grief dragging at their heels behind them.

*

Death came to each of those families like a bolt out of the blue: here today, gone tomorrow, no chance to prepare. But there are times when death has been steadily approaching, maybe for years, and yet even in these situations – in the face of overwhelming chronic illness – you can still find yourself in the role of teller of truths. Teller of secrets already known.

It was almost midnight and I made my way up the back stairs to one of the general medical wards. The ward was quiet, apart from the occasional sound of a siren drifting in from outside. I had not passed another person on my journey there and, when I arrived, the lights were already off. When I pushed open the double doors into the ward, a healthcare assistant looked up from where she was sitting, documenting fluid balances at the nurses' station and, recognising my scrubs, sur-mised that I had come from intensive care. She pointed to a side-room at the end of the ward.

I had come to the ward at the request of the medic-al team to review a patient who was dying of chronic illness. He was sixty years old, and around his bed sat his wife, daughter, sister and father. I remember being immediately struck by the observation that his father looked both fitter and younger than him. I hadn't seen this patient before, but it was no feat of great wisdom for me to realise that this man had severe heart failure and enough other chronic conditions to mean that this downturn was probably a terminal event.

There were no spare chairs in the room and, not wanting to add further to his vulnerability, I hunkered down next to his bed, before I introduced myself to him. Saying his name, I asked him how he was feeling. His eyes focused somewhere in my direction and he whispered 'Hello', but unfortunately, as is too often the case, it was clear that I had met this patient at a time when he was just too ill to communicate at any length with me. When I had finished examining him, I sat with his family and asked them if they had ever discussed what he might want at a time like this – at a time when he was dying.

The answer was no and their expressions seemed to convey a sort of sad helplessness. I persevered, asking if they thought he knew from his illness that this was an increasingly likely possibility. I asked if they thought he knew he was that unwell. They looked at each other first, then they looked at me again, and it really seemed as though perhaps they felt some regret, as if they wanted to be able to answer me, but that was not their reality. And so they answered again that they did not know.

Chronic illness is tricky like that. As a doctor, I knew he was dying, but for patients and relatives there may be no abrupt trumpet call, no herald. Chronic illness often doesn't come with the same aplomb that something more high-profile like cancer might. Often, the dying just creeps up on people. They are surprised, and then I find myself in this sort of moment: breaking news to people, telling them truths that have been known for a long time, and yet for some reason have remained inaccessible to them up until that point.

I phoned the consultant at home; he agreed, from what I told him, that this patient was going to die anyway, but said he would leave it to me to speak to the family again, and that a trial non-invasive ventilation was something I could offer them, if I felt it was appropriate. At this point the patient was struggling to breathe. He had had access to extra oxygen via a facemask on the ward, but it wasn't sufficient, and in these situations there can be an option to try non-invasive

ventilation. The 'non-invasive' bit means there is no tracheal tube involved, no tracheostomy. The patient needs
to be 'awake' and breathing for themselves, but we use
pressure to give them some help. The common options
for this are a mask that is strapped tightly around the
face to form a seal, or a hood that goes over the head like
a bubble and tightens at the base of the neck.

When I explain to people what non-invasive ventilation is, I generally try to be honest about what it
feels like. I tell them that wearing the mask might
feel like trying to breathe with your head stuck out
the car window on the way down a motorway, but
that if they can relax, most people get used to it. I
tell them that it can feel very warm inside the hood,
but I remind patients that they are always free to ask
us to stop – that they will be in charge. Every time
I have this conversation, a memory comes back to
me from long before it was my job to explain to patients how these things work. I was still in my first
year as a doctor and was working on a surgical ward,
when our team referred a patient to intensive care
for non-invasive ventilation via the hood device. It
did the trick, but when he got well enough to return

to the surgical ward before eventually going home, he was angry and said, with some apparent venom and through gritted teeth, 'You dressed me up in a hood like a clown. I'm never going there again.' Non-invasive ventilation isn't comfortable, and it isn't for everyone.

Pushing this memory from my mind, I presented the family with this option, making it clear to them that this was the only shot we had. If this option failed, we would not put the patient on a ventilator. If his heart stopped, we would not try and restart it; there would be no sense in that. His father had such a kind face. He placed his hand on my forearm, then squeezed it and said, 'I know you will bring me good news.'

I wished this were true. I knew that I would never bring him good news.

You might ask why then I had even agreed to take this patient to intensive care in the first place? Really, I was more sure than not that this patient was going to die. Perhaps I was not confident enough in my seniority to be absolute, but what I *was* absolutely sure about was that the family needed to see this stage fail. They need-ed to see the options shut down. His father had looked at me through his kind eyes, and my management plan in the wake of this felt defined by shades of grey. So I was treating the family as much as I was treating the patient; treating them as a unit.

The family sat with him in intensive care and I gradually spoon-fed them reality. Two hours ticked by, and I had clinical evidence that a trial of non-invasive ventilation had definitively failed to improve his immediate prognosis. We sat down together for the third time that night and I told them this was it. I explained that the right thing for me to do now was to make him comfortable as he died. You really do have to say the words at times like this: dead, death, dying. You have to say them clearly. Tears flowed down his father's cheeks as he told me that his son had promised that he wouldn't die first. When I heard those words I knew that perhaps this slow, creeping dying wasn't really a secret at all. There had indeed been some sort of conversation.

Then his father takes my forearm again. He looks at me imploringly, and asks if half an hour more might help, but in that instant things are black-and-white and I am standing on a line that is hard and fast. I think about my patient – the most important person in this equation – and, keeping his hand in mine, I tell his father: no, he is dying now. I am kind, but resolute. I play my part and break the news.

Do I sound cold? If I call myself a player, a device in their storyline, it is not out of disrespect. I am not dismissive of the enormity of what these people are facing. I do not seek to diminish it; be in no doubt that my patient, their family and their grief are the most important things in the room. Even if there are times when I might say that I feel emptiness, trust me when I tell you that emptiness is most definitely still a feeling. The bottom line has to be that I have a job to do, and I cannot do it if I am falling apart. Doing my job is the only good that I have to contribute to their situation.

But knowing how much to give of yourself to a situation is something you have to learn as you go along, and I am still learning. Not long ago, a young woman was brought into hospital with bacterial meningitis. It was a textbook presentation, an instant diagnosis, and so she was treated immediately, but she was already only semi-conscious when the paramedics rolled her into the resus department. Her temperature was higher than any I have ever seen, her heart was running a marathon. Everything we could do was done, but within three hours I pulled back the skin of each of her eyelids sequentially, to find that her pupils had become fixed and dilated. They had expanded to the size of five-pence pieces and, when I stared into those black, non-reactive holes, it was clear we had as good as lost the battle. It was never a fair fight to begin with.

The patient came to intensive care anyway, and the following morning her brainstem was dead. Brainstem death is a difficult concept. It happens when the structures at the base of your brain swell within the rigidity of your skull and then cease to function. Without a functional brainstem, you have no potential to be conscious, no potential to tell yourself to breathe or to regulate your body's systems appropriately. Your brain loses the potential to send messages to the rest of your body, and you cannot then know life, in any common sense of the word.

This patient's brainstem had died and so we took her family on a journey. Different consultants fed them the information they needed to know at different times. There was a predictable build-up and I was there most of the time, sometimes on the edges, sometimes at the front.

I was behind the head of the trolley, fiddling with the infusion pumps, when the nurse first guided the family in to see the patient in resus. I explained what the various tubes and drips were, and told them not to worry about the occasional alarms from the portable ventilator to which she was hooked up. I was the one who helped the emergency-department nurse wheel her round to intensive care, and who silently approached the chart to check progress over the next few hours. The next morning I came to break the news that the first set of tests had confirmed brainstem death, and afterwards I silently carried out the tests for a second time with the consultant as he narrated each step, when the family came to watch for themselves. They came to see what we called death, to try and understand it.

Even if I had been largely silent, I was around, so I presume my face became familiar. At least as familiar as you can be to a family who have found themselves lost in a nightmare unfolding rapidly over forty-eight hours.

The woman's mother was the personification of kindness. She put her arm around my back, she thanked

me a lot and she hugged me. When, on several occasions, she asked if there had been any change in her
daughter's response to treatment and I told her no, she
would touch her forehead gently to mine and whisper,
'Thank you for telling me, anyway.'

As I write this event in retrospect, I wonder if I should
find it odd that I would have such an intimate and close
exchange with a stranger, that I would accept that ges-
ture, or that she would even want to touch her forehead
to mine and it would not seem strange or misplaced to
me. In this job there are moments when the room is already full of strange and horrible truths, cruel twists of
fate and untimely endings, and I think in those moments
there is enough strangeness spinning around that there
seems no sense in heeding the rules of social engagement
that we reserve for those people we call strangers.

Her sister sat by the bed for hours, with her legs
pulled up to her chest. She was an adult, but still slight
enough that she looked lost and child-like. When, the
previous day, I had met her in the emergency department for the first time, she had also hugged me.

This family made the decision to consent to organ
donation, and when the time came for them to leave

their loved one behind in the hospital, they hugged me
again. There were a lot of hugs across those two shifts.
I don't mind. When you work in intensive care, it rapidly becomes clear that different families need different
things from a doctor. Sometimes they even need different things from different doctors on the same team. If
I am to be the one confronting them with that sort of
horror, I would rather be approachable. I would rather
appear kind. I would rather be the person they feel they
can hug, if that is what they need me to be.

There is a question, though, that I haven't quite
worked out the answer to yet: what do *I* need?

When a patient's relative hugs me through their sorrow, when they put their arms around me and create
that bond, even if it is just for a moment, do I expose
myself to a bit more of their pain? Does it make it harder to achieve the distance that lets you move on to the
next patient, and the one after that?

People who work in radiology wear dosimeters on
their lapels, small badges that act as a safety net to help
them recognise whether their cumulative exposure to
radiation is within safe limits. I can't help but wonder
what my grief-dosimeter might read. Does the dose I

receive increase when I am hugged? Does it climb when I become the vehicle of continuity in the short course of a family's painful journey? Do we even know what is a safe limit at all?

It is interesting to consider the true scope of what can become a normal part of your everyday working life: the list of things we say you get used to. As healthcare professionals, it often seems like a mark of strength that we can hold up – a defence. We tell ourselves that we are resilient, and really we are, because what is the alternative?

There are already occasions that I could look back at now and almost nostalgically label as rites of passage: the first time you verify a death; the first time you tell a family to prepare for the worst; or the first time you realise someone is going to die alone. The first occasion I became aware that an elderly lady was going to die alone, without any family or friends with her, I had been qualified for less than a month. I remember sitting in my car after work, still in the car park, phoning my mam at home and crying; sobbing about how sad I was, how sad it was that this woman seemed alone in this world and had no family, and nobody to be with her at the end.

My mam is a nurse, and so she's a good person to talk to in this kind of situation. She told me that yes, it was sad, but this patient would be cared for by the nurses and they would look after her, and I had looked after her; and these things matter too, that all of that counts for something. She told me those words in the same way she had told me not to be afraid of the dark when I was five; or when I was seven and found myself enthralled watching Freddy Mercury on television, commanding a stage with his crimson cape, and she told me that he had just died of AIDS: and yes, it was very sad, but he would be remembered for ever as a superstar, a phenomenon.

Here I was, all grown up, and I still needed her to tell me something beautiful. At this stage in my career I don't expect to cry about these things any more. There have been so many since then, how would I ever be able to? That sort of feeling isn't sustainable.

I try to focus more now on what it is that I can do for a patient who is facing the end without any loved ones around them. One morning, when I was three years qualified and working on a medical ward, I arrived at work a little early. I had planned to catch up on some preparation for ward-round, but I spotted one of my patients in the corner. He was ninety-four years old and tall, but thin and forlorn, with ribs that were visible through the material of his hospital gown. I had by this time looked after him for about a week, and now he was clearly in his final hours, grappling with his gown, tugging at it like he did not know how all of this had come upon him.

When I approached the bed, I sat and took his hand. I said his name and told him he was all right, because it is all I could think to say. He was quiet then and his two hands wrapped themselves around mine: bones drenched in skin. The medical students arrived on the ward enthusiastically, and asked me if they could help me prepare for ward-round. I replied that I wasn't sure when I would be free, and perhaps they could just get started.

Around me, the healthcare assistants washed and dressed their patients. The nurse with the drugs trolley was doing her morning round. The students made notes of the observations and blood results for the ward-round, and I remember making a mental note not to forget that I had some discharge letters still to release, after I was finished here.

I sat still by my patient. I stared at him and he stared at me. I wondered if he was really looking at me, or just through me. Perhaps he was looking at the face of somebody else that he had known before. As I sat there, I went through in my head the only words I have ever known to soothe myself in situations like this. They come from Raymond Carver:

> And did you get what
> you wanted from this life, even so?
> I did.
> And what did you want?
> To call myself beloved, to feel myself
> beloved on the earth.

I say these words in my head like a mantra, and I hope that the patient knew love or that they at least feel love in that moment at the end. Those words are the shield I have made for moments like that. The shield is for me. It helps me believe that what I can do in those moments counts for something.

Just twenty minutes passed like this before he died. I closed his eyes, verified his death and wrote in the notes his cause of death: 1a Sepsis, 1b Pneumonia, 2 Frailty. Then I found the medical students and started the routine of our morning reviews: 'Hello, Mr Smith, how are you feeling this morning? Did you manage to eat your breakfast?'

The patient's family had been informed, but they never came.

When relatives and friends grieve for their loved ones, they grieve for that patient: who they were and what they meant to their lives. When doctors find themselves unexpectedly ambushed by grief over the death of a patient, I think it is often for another reason. Yes, it is because that person could be our child, our friend, our brother, but it is often because that life didn't follow the rules of whatever vague, illogical structure we use to hold together our shaky universe. It is because they remind us of how little we can really control.

There was the patient who was thrown off his motorcycle into the road. The accident happened because a fox had run across his path and he had swerved to miss the animal. He arrived in resus and had the benefit of everything a modern major trauma centre had to offer. We gave him literally everything we had, and we still couldn't keep him alive. When I stood behind the curtain at his bedside to verify his death, I felt ambushed. I was surrounded by the fruit of decades of medical advances in intensive care and here was this man dead in the bed in front of me, because a fox had crossed the road. It just seemed so absurd, so meaningless. I listened for the absence of heart sounds and whispered a meagre apology: 'I'm so sorry we couldn't save you.'

Major trauma has made up a large number of the patients I have cared for in my training to date. Many of these patients will require a tracheostomy as part of their journey. This is a hole at the front of the neck that allows us to put a tube through it and down into the trachea. In intensive care there are different types of patients who, for one reason or another, might take some time being weaned from the assistance of a ventilator. A tracheostomy tube in these situations enables us to wake a patient up, without having to keep the endotracheal tube that goes through their mouth into the trachea.

Decannulation is what we call it when we make the decision to take the tracheostomy tube out. It is a word that really describes taking something away, but the day that tube comes out is about something else entirely. When you work in intensive care, decannulation day is about handing something back: go forth and breathe by yourself, expand your lungs and feel the air enter you in the way it was always supposed to; feel your breath flow over your vocal cords and remember that you have a voice that is all your own. It is about a surge of hope.

Putting in a tracheostomy is a different feeling. The patient lies sedated and flat, with their head extended backwards. You start by orientating yourself to a specific soft spot on their trachea called the cricothyroid membrane, then you work your fingers down the neck and pick a spot about halfway between that membrane and the top of their sternum.

When you've picked the point, you take your needle and pierce it through the trachea. When you guide the plunger of your syringe backwards and watch the air bubbles enter it, you know you're in the right place. Then you remove the syringe and feed a wire down through the needle. The wire goes right down into the lungs, to where the trachea splits to become the left and right main bronchus. Then you take the needle away and the next job is to dilate the hole around that wire, so that it becomes large enough to fit a tracheostomy tube through it.

It takes a lot of pressure to force something blunt through the skin and into the trachea, because its walls were made to stand apart, strong and full of air. But we have our tools; the brand of dilators that I have been taught to use is named after the horn of rhinoceros, exactly because they resemble that animal's defence equipment. You pick them up and direct your force down through the neck into the bed: short stubby dilator, then large dilator, followed by third dilator with the tracheostomy tube.

In the main, it is possible to do this procedure with little blood loss, but if you have trouble or nick a vein, blood rushes out around the hole in the trachea, creating a crimson geyser of air and blood. When I did a tracheostomy for the first time, it was a force that felt barbaric. The patient didn't feel it, but I did.

Then the day comes when you get to feel what it's like to take the tube out again.

There was a young patient who had been involved in a road-traffic accident on the motorway. She had been a student in her first year of university when the collision happened. Now she had progressed a long way in her slow recovery from this major trauma, and the physiotherapist had come to tell me that she felt today was the day our patient was ready for decannulation. She started first of all with a speaking valve and we gave her back her voice. Trying to speak is difficult at first, because the sound comes out raspy and quiet. It is more air than sound, more breath than words. This patient got her voice back and her first words were 'Thank you'. She said thank you to the physiotherapist and 'Thank you all so much.'

Then we took the tracheostomy tube out, and suddenly it felt like we could talk about the future. That moment makes you feel they have made it. It gives you permission to feel something hopeful. To really consider what the patient has to look forward to. Sitting out in a chair, she became something hopeful. Her friends came to visit and they looked comfortable, as if they once again knew how to relate to her. I beamed at the other staff on the unit: 'Have you seen her? We've taken the trachy out – doesn't she look great?' Decannulation day is just like that; it's a sort of celebration.

That patient died a week later. It was an unexpected death, unrelated to her tracheostomy or lack of it. I stood in disbelief. At work, I rarely stand in disbelief. Things may be sad, but I believe them. I verified her death and wrote it in the notes:

Time of death as verified.

Rest in peace.

Then I walked around the unit, and eventually into the charge nurses' office and said I was going to sit for a minute. The rest of the junior doctors had recently rotated to new jobs and I hardly knew the new team. The nurses were familiar, though, so I slipped inside their office and perched on a counter by the window. They didn't ask me why I was there, because they already knew; and then the charge nurse stood up and gave me a hug, and for the first time in years I cried at work. I sobbed in his arms for a minute and cried as if I did not know any better.

I cried because she was *supposed* to be okay, because I was screaming inside, 'These aren't the rules!' We took out the tracheostomy tube; she was going to be okay.

That is how I think grief most commonly visits me now: as an unexpected ambush, just when I am bold enough to believe I might have figured out – or even started to feel comfortable in – the world of critical care and illness in which I spend most of my days.

Much of medicine is high-stakes activity, because even the most benign tasks done incorrectly have the potential to adversely affect somebody's life. As a doctor, you learn to deal with this without any real advice or instruction; be on your guard, be mindful about what you're doing, but be rational. It is in nobody's interest for a doctor to spend their entire career in medicine with their stress levels chronically raised, so eventually we all end up coding – as routine – tasks that may once have seemed stressful. Routines don't always go to plan, though, and from this comes another type of grief that I have known in practice. I think I first realised that it *was* grief when I listened to a story from a consultant. His experience filled the room, and the air was thick with respect for what he had laid in front of us. He talked about 'the shadows that walk with us, the scars that make us who we are'. He was talking about making clinical mistakes. Mistakes are often difficult for doctors to talk about, but I would like to tell you about one of my own.

When I was almost four years qualified and working on a general medical ward, I looked at a chest X-ray for less than ten seconds, closed it and wrote in the notes: 'Chest X-ray – no evidence of pneumonia.' I was on-call that evening and was reviewing a man with multiple chronic illnesses, about whom the house-officer was worried. His septic screen had returned a mixed growth of bacteria in his urine, but despite five days of the appropriate antibiotics, he remained pyrexial and his inflammatory markers climbed.* The house-officer had

---

* A 'septic screen' is the process of casting a net to look for evidence of infection in blood, urine, any other available body fluid or with imaging, such as a chest X-ray. 'Pyrexial' is used to describe the state of having an abnormally high fever. 'Inflammatory markers' are substances in the blood, usually proteins, which become raised when there is any sort of inflammation in the body, including infection.

one of those 'This isn't quite right' feelings, but couldn't put his finger on what was wrong, so he had asked me to take a look.

I will not go into more clinical detail, because it took me a long time to be able to say that I made a mistake and then stop the sentence. It took me a long time not to mention all the other people who saw that chest X-ray, too, and all the other holes in the cheese. Even as they read this now, there will be doctors coming to their own conclusions about what I did or didn't do. Doctors have always been very good at judging each other, but for now you will have to be content with knowing that due process occurred, and the clinical details of this mistake were discussed in the proper forum at the proper time.

What I will tell you, though, is that three days later this patient became very unstable and developed shock. We discovered a perforation in his bowel. My heart raced when I sat at the computer to pull up that chest X-ray. I stared at the computer screen, waiting, knowing that I was about to be confronted with what I did not want to see. There was air under the diaphragm, the classic sign that something in the abdomen had perforated, and it glared back at me menacingly, because of course now I could see it and everyone else could see it – and how could anyone have missed it?

But I did miss it. Common and clichéd: my mistake of inattentional blindness. It's what you do when you look at an image for one specific reason. It's what happens when I show you a photograph and ask you to count the number of birds in the sky, and you do it, without spotting that the house on the hill is on fire. If I'd asked you instead to tell me about everything in that photo, you'd have spotted the house and you'd have said it was on fire.

Of course I told the consultant my truth: that I had looked at this chest X-ray three days before and had missed this sign. He looked at me earnestly and said, 'This is not your fault. You looked at it and you missed it. You missed it honestly, it was a mistake.'

Progressing in medicine is, in general, a bit like growing up; there's a growing realisation that you are important and, if you're lucky, what you do matters to more people than just you. The more senior you become, the more responsibility you acquire. The thing about responsibility is that if you take it as seriously as you should, somebody telling you that it wasn't *all* your fault doesn't really help you to deal with it. It is hard to take the get-out-of-jail-free card, and it gets harder to tell yourself those sorts of bedtime stories.

I carried that mistake around alone: heavy on my chest and close around my throat. I hardly knew what to do with it. There were days when I really tried not to think about it, but even on those days it was always there, still and looming as the reason I was afraid to think about anything at all. After some days I knocked on that same consultant's door. I remember him looking up from his desk at me as I said, 'I just can't stop thinking about it.'

Instinctively he knew exactly what 'it' was. I sat down and he told me that I must always be brave and responsible enough to look at and examine my mistakes honestly; but that is not the same as punishing yourself. He told me about the risk that comes with increasing seniority in medicine, and then he told me about his own mistakes, and I no longer felt so alone.

I think that working through a mistake remains the closest thing to real grief that I have ever experienced in clinical practice. When it comes to mistakes, people like to say, 'There's no use crying over spilt milk', but

I disagree, and I would venture that these people never made a mistake that impacted upon a life. There has to be a time for owning that sorrow, just as there is a time for pulling yourself together and owning the way you choose to get back up. I can't say it was easy, but I can say that getting to a place where I could look square in the face at the mistake I made and accept it, without falling, I felt stronger, and I felt in the end that it was the least I could do for that patient.

That patient died, as multiple other senior colleagues said that he would have done, either way; and, honestly, I believe and know they are right. Still, maybe I could have bought him one more day. Maybe he could have been told that he was dying, while he was still well enough to take it in. Maybe there was something he wanted to say to somebody close to him; and, crucially, maybe his family might have experienced a different sense of control and peace over the death of the person they loved.

The reality is that I will never know; grief happens, we accept it and somehow things move on.

Joy

I do not miss childhood, but I miss the way I took pleasure in small things, even as greater things crumbled. I could not control the world I was in, could not walk away from things or people or moments that hurt, but I took joy in the things that made me happy.

Neil Gaiman, *The Ocean at the End of the Lane*

PEOPLE ASK ME ALL the time if I 'like' my job. I always answer people the same: that despite not loving every moment of every day, I do love my job at least once a day, every day, and I think this makes me pretty lucky. Usually that kind of moment comes to me on a staircase while I am alone and on my way to a referral. It is something that is not rooted in one particular patient or achievement that day. It is just a realisation – a feeling that I might be in exactly the right place – and that feeling has become a great friend to me. It is an encounter like the subtle waft of air that makes you notice the smell of freshly cut grass in the summer time.

Joy, within the context of intensive-care medicine, doesn't always take form in the way you might imagine. But it is there. I know it is, because my work is often what gets me out of bed in the morning, and I can easily occupy a vantage point that enables me to appreciate immense worth in what we do. Nevertheless, the happiness that is eventually realised is rarely about unexpected moments of good fortune. It's not like running down the stairs on Christmas morning to find everything you asked for. It's not about winning an award, sealing a deal or bagging a big contract. It's not about fanfare. Finding joy in simple moments is therefore immensely important to me. Ultimately, the joy I can recoup from the work I do is most often about looking back on the ebb and flow of a patient's journey and recognising that, although their struggle will, most likely, have continued long after their discharge from the intensive-care unit, in the end there was probably some 'good'. And I think I have to be happy with this.

I have often considered that much of what I experience as joy at work is probably, in fact, pure relief. In intensive care we are presented with so much horror, and work under conditions of such uncertainty, that the relief that comes from knowing even a small part of a patient's recovery can be electrifying.

One evening I was standing at the end of a bed that I had stood at before. A month earlier I had watched this man lying somewhat contorted, slightly too tall for the bed, with his mouth hanging open and his tongue white from the insult of what his body had been through. There is something synonymous with death and those who lie with their mouth hanging open – it is as if they cannot bring themselves to close it. As if it hangs there, wide open, because they have become so separated from their presence in the room that it no longer matters to them. Doctors light-heartedly refer to this open-mouthed expression as the 'O sign', and it means that someone is probably 'on their way'. I had watched this man's eyes, wide too and tormented, yet entirely vacant, seeing everything but at the same time seeing absolutely nothing. I had felt his skin – wet, clammy and cold. It was the sort of eerie, sweaty cold that feels like someone has reached that temperature from the inside out. I had touched a man falling apart.

The awfulness and horror of watching someone lying like that, for days, is important here, because I want you to understand exactly why saying goodnight to somebody (whose surname you only really know because it is printed on the notes that you hold in your hand) can, in time, be responsible for so much joy.

A month later I am standing at the end of his bed and I notice his eyes participate in the smile that I am greeted with. Creases form at their corners. They are lines that prove not only that he has been happy many times before, but that he might be happy now. I pick up the TV remote control, because it was placed just out of his reach, and as I am leaving I say goodnight. In my head, his expression is a sign that he knows what I am thinking. That he can hear me think: thank you for getting better, for sitting up in bed and smiling at me like that. When I hand him the remote control, my fingers momentarily touch his hand and it is warm.

It is my experience that this is not the sort of joy my colleagues routinely share with each other. I might say, 'How great is it that Paul has started to make good amounts of urine again? His kidneys must be recovering.' I don't think I have ever said out loud, 'I looked at

Paul today and felt such joy; he seemed so far away from that man we watched disintegrating in a bed last month.'

Sharing that sort of feeling isn't really the 'done thing'. It remains a mystery to me why – particularly among adults who are privy to the view of the human condition that doctors have – this should be the case. The team that I work in is probably the most important determinant of how happy I can be, within the context of a day. The camaraderie required to be a successful team in the emergency specialities is paramount. The consultants I meet say that the most beneficial thing you can do to secure your happiness is to choose your colleagues wisely, and appreciate them. After all, we share the sort of emotional moments with our colleagues in this job that might usually be reserved only for close friends and family. So while it might not be common for me to sit and discuss the sort of joy I find in smiling at a patient, we do hold each other up in other ways. I can remember shutting the door of the office behind me, after a particularly difficult and emotionally stressful family conversation, to find another registrar waiting with a coffee and some cake. He said, 'You need this' and took my on-call bleep, so that I had time to decompress. It is to my advantage that I do not hold too many memories of traumatic and harrowing events that, thanks to my colleagues, aren't also memories of camaraderie and kindness.

I think people presume that at some point I also develop a relationship with most of my patients, and eventually benefit from the feedback this interaction creates. Apart from the occasional exception, I don't know if you can call what happens between doctors and patients in intensive care 'a relationship', in any true sense of the word. It is difficult to explain to someone how significant a patient and their journey can be in your life, when you do not know each other at all. Sometimes patients come back to visit intensive care, to see the place where it happened. It is a joy to look up from my work and see a former patient standing unexpectedly across the floor, sometimes barely recognisable to me in their recovered state. It's a joy that makes you exhale a warmth that runs up from your lungs and into your smile. But it is also entirely normal for me to have to introduce myself to a patient on that day. I greet them as if seeing them standing there is the most beautiful thing I have seen all day, even if they have absolutely no idea who I am. Many of the patients I meet will never know about the times I stood over them, about the conversations I had on their behalf or the time I spent engaged in trying to do the right thing for them.

I can recall the horror of a young woman screaming from her bed in intensive care. She was wailing, like a banshee, with the emotional pain and frustration that come from being so weak that she could no longer even swallow her own saliva effectively. She had every right to be angry, to scream and cry out. I often wonder why more patients don't do the same. This woman had every right to rail against the universe that had done this to her, and at the same time to long with every fibre of her being to be a part of it again. Her screaming filled every corner of the unit, the night that it started. It filled every corner of my brain and I was horrified, but not because I felt exactly what she felt. While I felt absolutely a deep sense of compassion towards her, of course I could only ever imagine that level of frustration. The horror came from feeling as if I was some sort of guard, complicit in the orchestration of her torment. Part of me wished she would not scream, because I knew I could not make her torment go away; another part of me wished the same thing, just so that I did not have to hear her scream. She was calmed in the end by a nurse, who took from her pocket a tube of scented hand cream and rubbed it slowly into each of her hands.

A few months later I was hurrying through the waiting room on my way to A&E when the same nurse said, 'Are you just going to walk past her?' I stopped and looked round at a young woman, smiling and with a toddler holding her hand. She stood there, one mother and her child, and it took me some seconds to see in her the same woman I had looked after for so long. It didn't matter to me that she would hardly know me as a significant part of her journey. Most of the care I gave her was received while she was not in a position to know that it was being given. It didn't diminish the joy.

The encounters that I 'share' with a patient are often not really shared by that patient at all. I spend my time in a seemingly infinite number of exchanges with humans, and create so many memories that will never be tethered within the consciousness of the other person. Often they exist within my head alone and, being only obligated to my own reality, I'm never sure what it is that they become, or can ever mean. I introduced myself to that patient-returned and told her how well she looked. Then I scooped up the joy that had been unexpectedly placed in my path that morning and carried it around for the rest of the day. There was joy, and there was relief in knowing that I now had another memory to soothe one of her screams.

In her poem 'Of Tolling Bell I Ask the Cause', Emily Dickinson wrote 'That bells should joyful ring to tell, A soul had gone to heaven'. I think I see too much death to believe comfortably in platitudes or generalisations. I understand that they have their place, that humans have a need to find a higher meaning in things, but on the whole I am no longer sure if I have that sort of conviction in any religious faith. But irrespective of whether or not you believe in heaven, death is an event just as connected to life as living is. Death is a life event that cannot be written off as something to be ignored until the last moment or swept under the carpet. Put simply: if you want to live, you have to die.

For some people, death comes abruptly, cruelly and without rhyme or reason. For others, it comes at the end of many years, and we might say that it is natural. For many, it is something in between. Whatever the scenario, death is a huge part of my job, and I think it would be impractical of me not to look for the joy that may come from working positively with those who are dying, just as I do with those who are surviving. I don't think you have to have an unshakable conviction in a higher being to find joy in death.

Finding joy in caring for a dying patient means meeting death head-on. You can't try to confront death from behind a cushion, with your head peeking out. You can't be avoidant, because death doesn't wait and doesn't care if you miss the opportunity to appreciate the moment.

Diana was a woman in her eighties who had been on the intensive-care unit for a little under a week. She had a history of coronary heart disease and had come to hospital with some further ischaemic damage to her heart.* It had given her end-stage heart failure, and her

---

* The coronary arteries are responsible for supplying the heart muscle with the oxygenated blood it needs to work effectively. In coronary heart disease, these vessels become blocked by deposits of atheroma or fatty material, formed in part by a build-up of cholesterol, and the blood supply to the heart's muscle becomes impaired. We call the damage 'ischaemic' when it occurs as result of inadequate blood supply.

only feasible chance for relatively short-term survival was some targeted medical treatment and non-invasive ventilation. I had looked after Diana for my previous two night shifts and, unfortunately, she hadn't really progressed. Now it was partway through night three and she had subtly started to declare herself as getting worse.

Diana lay in bed, sweating beneath the non-invasive ventilation mask, and her agitation came and went. Beneath that sort of mask it is often difficult to see a face that you can relate to; the mask becomes so overbearing. That night shift had been very busy for referrals. Diana's nurse recognised the slow creep of demise, and each time I walked past she showed me the results of a blood-gas measurement, to which I replied with something like, 'She's already at the ceiling of what we can do. If she starts to really decline, we'll make some decisions.'

The night ticked on. Another referral, another pitstop in between, to see how much closer Diana had inched to the cliff-edge. By the time 5 a.m. came, the nurse had started to see runs of non-sustained arrhythmia on Diana's cardiac monitor. She showed me another blood-gas measurement and gave me a look that warned me not to avoid the inevitable.

Aoife Abbey

I phoned the consultant and he agreed that we had reached the end of what we could provide, with a view to making Diana 'better', and that we should call the family in. I left the nurse to call them while I went to see another referral. When I returned, the family stood in vigil around the bedside, but I walked past, head down, because I was hurrying to another patient. Catching the nurse's eye, I pointed apologetically to my bleep and said, 'I'm sorry – five minutes.' She rolled her eyes pointedly.

Walking to the next patient, I wondered how I was ever going to present this woman with her choices. I do not consider myself uncomfortable with death as a topic of conversation, but there are aspects of it that are daunting. Speaking to a family about the impending death of their loved one can be routine, and even speaking to a patient about their thoughts for end-of-life care, which might become an issue weeks or months from now, rarely unnerves me. Sitting down to talk to a patient about their death, which is going to happen on this day and in this hour, that is something singular. The options for Diana were few:

100

Option 1: Accept that the non-invasive ventilation was already showing signs of failing, but
continue to use it over the next few hours, in the
knowledge that it was more likely than not that
she would die with the mask strapped to her face.

Option 2: Take off the mask and know that, in
doing this, she would die very quickly, probably
within minutes.

I wondered if I could justify holding off for three
hours, until the day shift. But I had nothing left on my
to-do list, nothing that I could convince myself was
more pressing. I met the family and explained that the
current treatment strategy wasn't working and I was
going to take Diana through her options. I knew it was
the right thing to do, but I wasn't sure if I knew exactly
the *right way* to do it. How do you tell somebody they
are going to die so imminently?

I sat down to talk to Diana, with the weight of the
family watching. She wanted them to stay. On the whole,
when it comes to having such a sensitive and important

conversation, the non-invasive ventilation mask is a hindrance. One helpful aspect, however, as I realised then, is that it means you really need to get quite close to the patient, so that you can hear each other above the noise of the machine and through the plastic that shields most of the patient's face from yours. I therefore sat close to Diana, with one hip on the bed; and, once I had started to speak, the rest of the room melted away.

Diana decided she wanted to take the mask off, and she asked me if we would have to send her somewhere else first. I told her no, she would stay with us. She asked me then if it would hurt, and I told her we would keep her very comfortable, that it would be quick and that her husband and children would be right beside her. When Diana and I had finished talking, I turned around to the family and a nurse, who were all crying. I had really forgotten they were still there at all.

The family spent some minutes together with Diana, before the mask came off. When the nurse reached for the straps of the mask, I had a sudden uncomfortable feeling of responsibility for that woman's death. Through rational eyes, I know that Diana's death had come at a time that was natural for her, and it wasn't my choice that she was dying. But I felt the weight of knowing that Diana would only die once, and of realising that how things played out in these minutes would stay with her family for ever. Sometimes I feel frustration as a doctor when it seems as if people forget that death is not my invention; it is not my puppet or plaything. But there was a second when I wondered: Am I doing the wrong thing?

Then the mask came off and Diana's face lit up. She gave a broad smile and said five words that will for ever be special to me: 'Ah, that is a relief.'

Relief had never sounded so onomatopoeic to me.

She asked for a drink and I filled a plastic beaker of water, then handed it to her husband, so that he could put the straw in her mouth. Then I left.

She died within five minutes.

'Ah, that is a relief'; Diana did not say those words for me, but I was immensely grateful to her for them. They gave me joy, in that moment. The joy and privilege of knowing that we had given her a chance to experience something other than pain and distress at the end of her life.

The day team came for handover. When we reached Diana's name on our list, nobody was surprised that she had died. Before I left, I thanked the nurse for helping me do the right thing. I got in my car to drive home and when I stopped, bleary-eyed, at a red light, I thanked Diana, too.

You might think that some of these examples are sad events to tie my joy to, because they can only be housed along with memories of anguish or grief. But if I set my threshold for joy on waiting around for events devoid of any prior pain or trauma, I would be waiting a long time. Intensive care is about lots of things, but it is not about defeating death and it has little to do with miracles.

I don't believe the sickest people that I meet throughout my day at work are in the business of having outlandish desires, either. I don't think they are staring at the square-tiled ceiling of the intensive-care unit and dreaming of being an astronaut or an explorer. I don't think they're holding the hand of their wife and thinking, 'I hope we win the lottery and become rich.' Perhaps I am wrong, but I think they are, for the most part, simply hoping they will get to be a part of life again. They are hoping for all the things we take for granted every day: the ability to breathe by yourself, to get out of bed, to sit on a toilet or lie in a bath. To swallow your food and choose what you want for breakfast. To walk out into the world and appreciate all its beauty, or complain about the weather – but to have that choice.

I have had the pleasure of looking after patients who come out the other side of organ transplants. One New Year's Eve I was talking to a woman who'd just had a heart-and-lung transplant. She was the only one of my patients who was still awake when the bells chimed. We brought her some of the orange juice that we had poured into plastic champagne flutes and, as my glass tipped hers, I asked her what it felt like to have new lungs.

I don't think she expected the question, but after pausing for a second or two, she told me that she had forgotten what it felt like to breathe deeply. I asked her where she felt she might most like to go when she got out of there. I remain surprised that, as often as I have asked this question, nobody has ever given me a wild ambition or desire.

'I don't know. I've been taking one day at a time for so long now.'

'Maybe the answer is wherever you want to be,' I suggested.

Then, having been prompted to think about it, she added that she might like to go to the beach. 'Even if it is cold,' she told me. 'It would be nice to be outside.'

In medicine, the imperative constantly staring you in the face is that the world you see is rarely about magic or miracles. It is rarely even about justice. As a doctor of seven years, I am probably already capable of being more cynical than the average person; I can be ruthlessly cynical, and it is a survival mechanism that has its place. Despite all my conscious efforts to remain levelheaded, however, there are some stories that I choose to try and extract some magic from. I hold on to them because I also believe, unashamedly, that cynicism is not the only way to get through the day.

It was 6 p.m. and I was on the last of five long day shifts. The consultant on-call for intensive care that day had an odd way of making me feel disapproved of. Throughout my shift I had felt like a disappointment. Everything I did seemed to be a little bit wrong, in his eyes, and there had followed waves of frustration, and of wondering if I was the right sort of doctor for this speciality at all.

The medical registrar had called to ask if I would come to resus to see a man in his late seventies with sepsis. George was an active man for his age, worked full-time in a voluntary capacity and had come in with his daughter, who sang in her local community choir. Following the usual clinical examination and review of his notes so far, I began to explain to them what sepsis was. I started by suggesting that perhaps they had already heard the word on the news, or in a campaign. When they indicated this was not the case, I went on to explain that, in sepsis, instead of just the part of your body where the infection starts being affected, your whole body decides to react. Your blood pressure becomes low and, although sometimes fluid helps initially, it would not be wise to keep giving a patient with sepsis intravenous fluid indefinitely, because that would create multiple problems of its own.

George's daughter now looked at her dad with stern kindness and said, 'So you won't be going to that meeting tomorrow – I don't want to hear any more about it;

isn't that right, *Doctor?*' I have come to realise over the years that people are most likely to refer to me as 'Doctor' when they want me to agree with them.

I did agree and explained that, in fact, I would like George to come to intensive care for a central venous line and some blood-pressure support, because I was worried that his blood pressure was now so low that he hadn't made any urine in the past few hours.*

As expected, George didn't seem overly enthusiastic, but his daughter chimed in again, trying to rejuvenate his spirit by reminding him that her choir was giving a concert in a few weeks. 'Come on, Dad,' she said. 'I'm singing "Fight Song" at the next concert! You said you would come, so you'll need to be better for that.'

I will probably regret admitting that 'Fight Song' is in fact my alarm tune; it wakes me up in the morning. For those of you who aren't well acquainted with it, it is a song co-written by singer Rachel Platten and

---

* A central venous line is a way of delivering drugs or fluid into one of the larger veins. As opposed to a peripheral cannula, which might go into your hand, a central line is longer and contains multiple lumens or lines; it goes into one of the internal jugular or subclavian veins near the neck, or into the femoral vein where it is accessible in the groin.

songwriter Dave Bassett, and the chorus runs: '*This is my fight song ... And I don't really care if nobody else believes, 'Cause I've still got a lot of fight left in me.*'

I relayed to George and his daughter this embarrassing fact and, before I knew it, we were all singing the chorus of 'Fight Song' together in the cubicle in resus. The blood-pressure cuff cycled again and George's systolic blood pressure had come up from 70 to 90mmHg. I smiled to myself and, knowingly ridiculous, considered that perhaps sepsis management could benefit from the odd outburst of song.

I left resus to arrange a bed for George and wondered on the way back what the disparaging consultant would have thought about my impromptu singalong and unorthodox treatment for hypotension. I came to the conclusion that I didn't care. And I guess that was *my* fight song.

I don't often sing at work, though I did once traverse a waiting room accidentally singing the 'Heigh-Ho' song from *Snow White and the Seven Dwarfs*, and I'll never forget the summer when one patient's constant singing left 'We Wish You a Merry Christmas' engrained in my brain for most of August.

'Help! help! help! help! ... Now bring us some figgy

pudding!' Rose half-bellowed, half-sung this from the bed in her side-room. Over and over. Day after day. In the beginning, I ran in and out of the room trying to figure out what danger she had been presented with. By now I had got used to it. Her calls floated around my head like the soundtrack to my day.

Rose had come to the gerontology ward first of all with an infected ulcer on her leg. This infection itself didn't take long to treat, but then her psychiatric issues took over and her intended short stay on our ward escalated into months of confinement. I was a new doctor then, fresh on the wards and still in my very first job.

Acute infection aside, nobody really knew what was wrong with Rose: advanced dementia, perhaps severe depression, behavioural issues, aggression. We went round and round with diagnoses, while her middle-class retired life faded away into the distance somewhere. Rose had been an accountant; now her husband hardly knew her, and the truth was that we hardly knew what was wrong.

We discussed her at a multidisciplinary meeting and they called for specialist psychiatric nursing-home

care. Suitable places were few and far between, however, so Rose continued to wait, and more than a month
passed. Sometimes she shouted. Sometimes she just lay
there, ignoring my questions completely. Occasionally
she would act entirely inanimate, play dead and wait
until I had timidly crept right up next to her head to
ask how she was, then let out an earth-shattering and
perfectly timed roar, to send me jumping into the air.
She didn't answer questions – nothing went both ways.
Every single interaction fell crashing between us onto
the floor.

One day, about eight weeks into Rose's time with
us, it was close to 5 p.m. and I was leaving her room.
'See you tomorrow, Rose,' I said habitually as I left,
but then I stopped. I had heard my name (she knew my
name?), followed by two words: 'I'm lonely.' I could
hardly believe my ears, and rushed to her bedside. 'I'm
sorry, do you want to talk?'

She didn't.

We could read a book, or the newspaper perhaps?
She asked me for a crossword.

For eight weeks we had done our utmost to care for
Rose. She had been washed, dressed and fed. We had

given her antibiotics and antipsychotics. We put cannulas in her veins and collected blood and urine for our
tests. We sought opinions from psychiatry, neurology
and gerontology. We wanted so much to help her, but
all our leads were dead ends. Rose herself had never
directly asked us for a single thing, but now she had
asked me for a crossword and I felt like I would have
walked over hot coals to bring one to her.

I bolted out of that room like I was looking for the
cardiac-arrest trolley. 'I need a crossword!' I called
out loudly, as I darted into the activities room to rifle
through a box of magazines.

The nurses gathered and peered through the little
side-room window in awe. This felt like Oliver Sacks's
Awakenings – the closest thing you might get to a miracle in care of the elderly. I sat on a chair by her bed and
found that Rose knew every answer in that crossword.
I just did the writing. I stayed in that room with her for
almost two hours and we spoke, back and forth, after all
those months as though nothing strange had ever gone
on between us.

The next morning, I opened her door with anticipation. 'Good morning, Rose.'

But there was no reply – Rose did not move or even look at me, and nothing more occurred between us again. She left us for a nursing home a few weeks later, whoever she was still locked away.

I sometimes think this might be the most exhilarating, joyous and yet simultaneously sad memory that I have of medicine. There isn't a perfect word to describe it, but perhaps it was bittersweet. When I sit every so often and think about what happened the day we did the crossword, it all still feels a bit like magic, and I am content to indulge myself and believe that is what it was.

You will know by now that I do a fair amount of what we call 'breaking bad news', but we don't actually have a formal expression for 'breaking' good news. To be honest, I find I rarely do it, and it doesn't require special study because as long as you are telling the truth, it is difficult to do good news badly. When news is truly good, it can frame itself. It isn't that good things don't happen on intensive care, it's just that when they do, they happen slowly: one marginally better day after another, so that recovery never seems like any great announcement. When W. B. Yeats dreamed about taking himself off to 'The Lake Isle of Innisfree' he said that 'peace comes dropping slow'. In intensive care, the truest thing I can say about good news is that, for the most part, it comes dropping slow. Good news is a collection of very tiny triumphs.

In the annual primary-school nativity play, my youngest sister was chosen to be the Angel Gabriel. She stood on the stage triumphantly and proclaimed, 'Do not be afraid! I bring you good news!' At five years old, I was given a much more low-key, non-speaking role. However, I have of late had the privilege of being an Angel Gabriel of another kind and it happened, too, at Christmas. I do understand that framing an event at Christmas is the sort of saccharine detail that might make a story less credible, but it is true, and I like to think of that as the universe's way of telling me to keep my burgeoning cynicism in check.

I wasn't looking for a Christmas miracle. Experience has taught me that whatever laws govern this planet that we share, they don't care if it's a holiday. At 2 p.m. on Christmas Eve a woman in her early sixties was brought into the resus department. She'd had a cardiac arrest at a shopping centre. As far as places to have a cardiac arrest go, this hadn't been the worst one; there was a nurse among the crowds of shoppers, there was a defibrillator and, importantly, she had a shockable heart rhythm. We received her in the emergency department with a regularly beating heart, so all that was left for us was to set about the usual process of stabilising her and carrying out the necessary post-cardiac-arrest workup.

Her family arrived: one son, a daughter-in-law and a ten-year-old grandchild. While we were all still in resus, another cardiac arrest arrived. I excused myself and helped the team deal with the newly arrived patient, behind the thin curtain right next to them. The other patient was an emaciated male who had just turned forty. He had long brown hair, a full beard, hollow cheeks and temples. His eyes were too big for his shrunken face, and his ribs stuck out from his naked torso. A more impractical person would not be shy to tell you that he looked like Jesus, taken down from the cross. He died shortly after arriving.

When I returned to the other family, the son asked, 'That person didn't make it, did they?'

Caught off-guard, I didn't know what to say. Thankfully, his wife stepped in with, 'Love, the doctor can't tell you that.' They knew the patient had died. But they didn't know he was exactly twenty years younger than their own relative.

The intensive-care consultant that day had asked me to attempt to wake and extubate her while we were still in the emergency department, and her son had asked if they could stay. I gave them the talk about patients not 'waking up' cleanly, as they might do on TV. I warned them that she might be agitated, that there would undoubtedly be some biting or coughing on the tube, that she might not recognise them at first. They insisted they wanted to stay and, as long as they were informed, I was happy to have them there, so I continued.

When the patient was seemingly alert enough, I pulled the tube out and watched her family wince. They turned away when I suctioned out her mouth. She was extremely agitated. I waited for it to pass, but it didn't. She was a tall woman and she writhed around on the trolley like a confused and angry bear. She pawed at her lines and made repeated attempts to lunge herself out of the bed. We transferred her to intensive care, but nothing in our arsenal settled her safely, so before I left that evening we made the decision to re-sedate and intubate her for the night. Her family left, deflated, with the grandson in tears. I remembered it was Christmas Eve.

The following morning I asked the nurse to stop the sedation first thing, and joked that I was pinning all of my happiness for Christmas Day on this woman waking up beautifully, this time around. And at 10.30 a.m. on Christmas Day I walked past the bed and she was sitting up in bed, talking to a nurse.

The family arrived half an hour later. 'How is she?' her son asked, holding his wife's hand, with the grandchild hovering behind them.

'Oh,' I said. 'Well, last time I saw her, she was having a cup of tea.'

'Are you joking?' exclaimed the grandchild.

'No,' I reassured him, 'I would never joke about that.'

I watched their faces, as the truth of this good news sunk in, and then watched them run down the intensive-care unit to where their mother and grandmother sat upright in bed on Christmas morning.

Let me be clear that her survival was not a miracle.
This was a case of a shockable heart rhythm and an early
defibrillation, in an otherwise fairly healthy female. It
was an expected positive outcome, and a testament to
exactly what bystander CPR and well-placed portable
cardiac defibrillators can achieve.

But that is not what this miracle was about. The
thing about this memory is that when I watched that
woman's family running towards her, I was miles away
from my own family. I was not able to go home or be
near any relatives for Christmas, and I would go home
to an empty house that evening. Yet I stood there and
was able to feel happier than I had ever expected to, at
work on that day. Their joy filled me up and, in that moment, it felt like a wonderful gift. It felt like something
I was supposed to take home, and one might be justified
in thinking that part really could be called a Christmas
miracle.

Me? I guess I am far too sensible for that.

Distraction

Distracted from distraction by distraction.

T. S. Eliot, *Four Quartets*

Feel for a pulse;

Asystole.

Epinephrine,

Compressions.

Feel for a pulse;

Asystole.

Compressions.

Feel for a pulse;

Asystole.

Epinephrine,

Compressions.

A YOUNG MAN HAD hanged himself and was brought to the emergency department in cardiac arrest. He had last been seen by his family a few hours before he had been found, and now he lay in front of me on a resuscitation trolley with bloodshot eyes, a ligature mark dug deeply into the side of his neck and the cardiac-arrest team buzzing around him. He was solid, with a chest that could take the weight and depth of the compressions that pounded up and down upon it.

There's a moment when his seemingly strong, muscular body makes me notice the stark contrast between his outward appearance and the despair that he now embodies. Then I remember it's this kind of thinking that leaves too many men unable to ask for help, and I wish very much that I had not thought it. I look at him and briefly recall the words of Stevie Smith:

> Nobody heard him, the dead man,
> But still he lay moaning:
> I was much further out than you thought
> And not waving but drowning.

Now focus, and CPR continues:

Feel for a pulse;

Asystole.

Compressions.

Feel for a pulse;

Asystole.

Epinephrine,

Compressions.

Feel for a pulse;

Asystole.

Compressions.

Asystole is what somebody in a film or on television might refer to as a 'flat-lining'. In reality, it is never actually a flat line that you see on the cardiac monitor, it is an ever so slightly wavy line that means the patient's heart is doing nothing useful. It is the bit in the TV show where the cardiac monitor goes: beep, beep, beep, beep, beeeeeeeeeeeeeep. Right now, in this real hospital, the team leader says that if the next rhythm is still asystole, we will stop. He moves his eyes around our group and asks if anyone present disagrees with that plan. We don't disagree.

But now it is ventricular fibrillation. The muscle fibres of this patient's ventricles have launched into an uncoordinated trembling and he still does not have an effective circulation, but as there is now some electrical activity, we seize the moment:

> *Shock,*
> Compressions.
> Feel for a pulse;
> Ventricular fibrillation.
> Shock,
> Compressions.
> Feel for a pulse;
> Ventricular fibrillation.
> Shock.
> Compressions.
> Epinephrine
> Amiodarone
> Feel for a pulse.

A pulse.

Are you sure?

Oh yes, I feel it too, here – tapping my fingers on his neck.

A pulse.

The poetry of CPR and a heart restarted. During those few minutes my attention is not properly focused on the details of the life I'm trying to save, not really. I am squeezing the ventilation bag, watching people pushing on his chest, calling time for a pulse check, asking if we had given adrenaline, and how many cycles is that now? We are taught to carry out cardiopulmonary resuscitation in a classroom by practising it over and over again on a hard plastic dummy. We learn the steps together like a dance, so that you don't have to think too much when the time comes. The correct rate of compressions is 100 times a minute; when I first learned CPR, we were told that you can make sure you hit the appropriate metre by thinking of a song. The one I use is 'Nelly the Elephant':

> *Nelly the elephant packed her trunk*
> *And said goodbye to the circus,*
> *Off she went with a trumpety trump;*
> *Trump, trump, trump.*

I still recite it in my head for the first dozen or so compressions, so I know I've got the metre right. If there is a student or a new junior doctor who is clearly a novice to real-life compressions and they're going too slow or too fast, I sing it quietly but out loud for them until they have got the right speed. Then I tell them they're doing great: just sixty seconds left, thirty seconds left, hang on in there, just ten seconds left. You'd be surprised how much a two-minute cycle of cardiac compressions can take out of you.

The song may seem incongruous with what you might expect the mood should be in that sort of situation, but its purpose is to ensure the patient receives 100 compressions a minute. Don't over-think it; a heart has stopped, and over-thinking is merely a distraction. For now, this is the time for dancing the dance.

Then the young man's pulse comes back and, as we set about doing some post-resuscitation workup, there is a pause; a lull in the intensity. People have often asked me how I cope with the pressure of this sort of situation. Recently, at the end of a thirteen-hour shift, I was confronted by a one-year-old whose heart stopped during our team's emergency intubation. My friends say, 'I don't know how you do it', and the simple answer is that I was trained to do it. We are all trained to move methodically through these moments. I don't tell them that nobody actually trains us for what happens next. They don't train us for the thoughts that come afterwards.

The pause would perhaps not be perceptible to those on the outside, but it is a break in which our routines become less choreographed. My mind wanders and I begin to imagine the patient's narrative. Now there is nothing to stop me from wondering what great sadness made him feel that hanging himself from a rope was better than living. I look down at his face and wonder if, from somewhere, he can perhaps see this stranger, with her hair high in a ponytail, wearing blue scrubs and pink-and-navy trainers, shining a torch into each of his fixed and dilated pupils. I wonder if we might ever have passed each other on the street before.

It is crucial to realise that restarting a heart is not the same as restarting a life. When a heart is young and healthy, I am not usually surprised to see evidence that the muscle has begun to contract, relax and beat again, eventually. Whether or not the patient will know 'life' again generally depends on how much oxygen their brain got while it was waiting for the circulation to come back. In the time it had taken for a family member to find the young man, the paramedics to get him down, start CPR, transport him and eventually for one of our team members to feel his pulse beneath their fingers, pushed into the crease of his groin, this young man's brain hadn't got enough oxygen. The subsequent CT scan of his brain made the approaching outcome clear to me. I knew we would soon be verifying his death, but there is due process and it doesn't do to jump ahead. I gathered his family and explained to them that it wasn't good news, that we would try and keep him stable over the course of the day and, later, we would check to see if his brainstem was still functioning. I told them that if his brainstem wasn't functioning, this would be equivalent to a verification of death. I told them this was the most likely outcome.

'But you think he still might wake up?'

'I have to be honest and say that no, I don't think he will.'

Hours tick by and the patient's brother approaches me alone, to ask if there has been any progress. I tell him no and reiterate that it is unlikely the patient will ever wake up. He says, 'I know what you're saying, but try getting them to believe it', and he gestures to where the mother and other brother now stand around the bed. I tell him they will believe it when they have to. For now, they have time for some distraction, and who am I to say it is not what they need?

Distraction is sometimes what people are compelled to seek while waiting for the inevitable, and I cannot brand that as cowardly or wrong. The musicians of the RMS *Titanic* continued to play their music even when it became evident that their ship was sinking. Three violinists, three cellists, a bassist and a pianist played their music amidst the horror of that night. All eight musicians went down with the ship, which led one second-class passenger to comment, 'Many brave things were done that night, but none were more brave than those.' When I stand back on the outside and watch a family sitting steadfastly around a bed, even when they have been told their ship is sinking, I think they are brave.

The benefit of distraction in the face of impending doom is, of course, not absolute. The correct balance is extremely tricky to achieve, and I have seen relatives waste away what seem like precious moments through their refusal to accept the reality that is staring them in the face. Relatives will, with predictable frequency, feel obliged to tell me their loved one is 'a fighter'. They never really come to me and say, 'You know what? He was more of a pacifist, actually. He was a bit lazy and he didn't really fight all that much.' I'm never sure if they're trying to convince me or themselves, but their own hope must have something to do with it. The concept of fighting something has become ingrained in the way our society feels about illness, and I have seen countless people distract themselves with that exact phrase, even in the face of expected and inevitable death.

One afternoon a father who was moments away from death was brought to hospital in an ambulance. He was clearly dying from terminal cancer, and one of his daughters was telling her dad to fight, that he *had* to fight. His son was arguing the same thing with the consultant, who was standing about a metre away from us. The consultant told the son that his dad *was* going to die now, and that we would do everything we could to keep him free from pain and comfortable, but that he should use this time to be with him. I pleaded the same thing with the daughter: 'This is an opportunity to be

with your dad; please think about using these minutes to be with him.'

During this encounter I stood squeezing a ventilation bag at the head of the trolley. Although this man was definitively and actively dying, there had been some confusion in the accuracy of information given to the paramedics. They hadn't been told he had a terminal condition – I presumed his family wanted there still to be some hope and so, when he arrived in resus, he did so with a laryngeal-mask airway in place and his heart was beating, but he was not conscious at all. I took over ventilation while we investigated and clarified what we could about the patient's background. It was soon clear that nothing we could do would change this man's fate and that I should stop artificially ventilating him.

But by this time the patient's family has arrived in the busy, open-plan resus department and what they see now is their dad, who is 'a fighter', and all they want me to do is keep squeezing that bag. They tell me that I have to keep squeezing the bag. 'You're not going to stop, are you?' Everything becomes about the bag. I could say, 'Yes, I am', but I know that they aren't ready. It takes the consultant another ten minutes to bring the family's focus round to the imminent death in the room. Eventually we see them connect with what is happening, and I look at the consultant with a face that says: 'Please, can I stop now?' The heart rate had slowed to near asystole and I feel intrusive in the scene of their goodbye. He nods at me and, because the time is right, the family does not notice my hand become still. I am not there. I slip out from behind the bed and leave through the curtain.

People often imagine death personified as the Grim Reaper. Distraction is not generally associated with a purpose, but if you stop and imagine distraction personified as a creature with a job to do, you might see that he is a surprisingly busy and prolific force in our world; what distraction chooses to touch fills up the trolleys in the emergency department all the time.

One day, distraction loomed over a teenager who'd been a pedestrian hit by a car. People allude to that sort of tragedy when they want an excuse to eat some cake or blow their wages on something unnecessary or expensive. They say, 'Hey, I could get hit by a bus tomorrow!'

and the people around them reply, 'Yeah, you're right, you could be dead tomorrow.' We say these things in jest, but that sort of event is also a reality. If I took a mental walk around the intensive-care unit I worked at that day, the roll call would have read:

> Pedestrian versus truck
> Pedestrian versus train
> Car versus tree
> Car versus truck
> Pedestrian versus car
> Bicycle versus car
> Fall from scaffold

One of those people had tried to end their own life. The rest of them were just going about the business they had set out for that day; they never saw death coming. Most of us exist in this state, where we take living for granted. We look left and right when we cross the road, mostly. We keep to the speed limit, except when we're late, and sometimes when the road is empty. We always wear a seat belt, except when we're not going that far. And we leave matters like talking about our feelings and wishes concerning organ donation until later.

When distraction visited this teenager hit by a car, we told her family that her brainstem was dead. The family said they still believed that she might wake up. 'It's what you do,' one person replied. 'We have to hope.' The family around her murmured assent, as if agreeing that this was to be their official battle strategy.

As I listened, the inexperience in me wanted to just say no: brainstem-dead means they will never 'wake up'. The focus on hope for some sort of miracle was an unwelcome distraction from the truth of their loved one's death, and from the potential option for organ donation. However, the consultant who was with me did not say that. He didn't dismiss the family or show any hint of frustration, but instead reiterated patiently the concept of brainstem death, before replying measuredly that if a miracle was going to happen, it would happen regardless of what we did next. It wasn't his job to argue against miracles.

Brainstem death often offers a unique opportunity to make the gift of life to others, but it is difficult to concede to organ donation when you can't concede to letting go of the final bit of hope that tells you your loved one might wake up. When a patient gives the gift of organs after brainstem death, they leave their relatives with a verification of death, but a heart that is still beating and a chest that is moved up and down by a ventilator. That this is what death *can* look like is not an insignificant concept to get your head around, even at the best of times; and when somebody you love is broken on a ventilator, your brain will be awash with hope and fear and grief. It is not the best of times.

We talked about organ donation, and although the patient in question had never ventured an opinion to her family on what she would have wanted, it transpired that their grandfather had received a deceased-donor liver transplant in the past. But the family still said no, and inwardly I found myself begrudging their decision. I was frustrated that they were so preoccupied with looking for a way out of this situation that they could not even consider the option that might save another life.

Later, when the patient's heart stopped and the ventilator was turned off, I heard the low sound of that family's sobs and watched their shadows as they stood around the bed, behind the paper curtains. I saw the pain in their eyes as, one by one, they walked off the unit and left this teenage girl behind, and I knew that I had never felt pain like it. Maybe holding out for a miracle had held them together; maybe it gave them something positive to focus on. And my focus on the opportunity to pay life forward to someone else had distracted me from the reality of their nightmare. A daughter was dead.

As a doctor, or indeed any healthcare professional, there is constant pressure to juggle tasks. Multitasking is in itself not unique to our profession, but when you deal in the lives of people, nobody wants to be the one who drops the ball. According to *Guinness World Records*, the longest time spent juggling three items without fail is twelve hours and five minutes. I have had shifts that last longer than twelve hours and five minutes. Thankfully in healthcare we work in teams, so if you're lucky somebody else will catch the ball for you. Hospitals are full of near-misses, some more serious than others. Frequently it is the considered questioning of a nurse that saves my juggling act:

'You've written milligrams here – did you mean micrograms?'

Between those words there is a 1,000-fold difference in the dose of a drug.

'You're not forgetting to see Mr Pearse, are you? He has had chest pain this morning.'

Yes, I had absolutely forgotten. Mr Pearse was having a heart attack.

Much of the time, a busy teaching hospital is full of competing interests. My tasks often include both teaching and learning, as well as treating the patient in front of me and being mindful of the other patients still on my list. One evening as a second-year doctor I was teaching two medical students who were shadowing me in the emergency department, while simultaneously prescribing drugs for a patient who'd had a heart attack. I wrote the wrong dose for one of the drugs. Thirty minutes later a friend of mine, who was a doctor on the ward where the patient had been sent, picked up the drug-kardex, saw my error and changed the dose. I had been distracted from that task by trying to teach the medical students – or was that task distracting me from teaching the medical students? Maybe I was doing both badly. I wondered if I had done that before. I wondered about the errors that people had seen and not told me about.

In medicine, we have a document called *Good Medical Practice*. It is essentially *the* rule book, issued by the General Medical Council, which is responsible for the licensing of doctors within the UK. The first rule is to 'Make the care of the patient your first concern'. It is of course the most natural thing in the world for a doctor to uphold this rule, but the truth is that sometimes it becomes a more deliberate thought-process than you would like. Sometimes I find myself being careful to make sure I have just the right focus – for example, when there are many patients in front of me, but limited time and resources to give them.

One winter night I was in the resus department with a young female who was unconscious, following an intentional overdose of prescription drugs. She had been intubated and ventilated to keep her alive. This particular week was a really busy week in a really busy winter. We'd been advised by bed management that the closest bed for her was forty miles away, but the sister on critical care phoned round the local units and eventually we negotiated a bed somewhat nearer. When her parents were told that our hospital didn't have a bed to accommodate their daughter, they were understandably upset, but the circumstances simply weren't appropriate to move any of our other patients. So they waited anxiously to be told where we could manage to fit her in. I watched the relief on their faces when they were finally told we had secured a bed and it was only ten miles away.

Meanwhile we had already been alerted to another critical patient less than ten minutes out, so the daytime registrar, who had already finished his shift, stayed on to transport to the other hospital the girl who'd taken an overdose. I scanned down the line of resus bays and registered that they were all full. The emergency-department consultant recognised my concerned look and assured me that they were moving one patient out to accommodate the incomer. I looked and saw that the healthcare assistant was packing up the chosen patient, so I helped her push them out of resus and round to the major-injuries unit.

We negotiated our way past rows of patients on trolleys in the corridor. 'Cubicle ten!' the coordinator called to us. But when we got to cubicle ten, it was already occupied with another patient. They were all occupied.

'I'll sort it out,' the coordinator assured me, so I left that patient with her and hurried back round to the resus department. The next patient was post-cardiac arrest, but he had been shocked back into a normal rhythm and stabilised, so we intubated him and got him ready for an urgent coronary angioplasty.* That angioplasty would save his life, and I should have been pleased with our teamwork, but when I handed him over to the anaesthetist in the catheter lab, my main concern was where we would find a bed for him when he came out the other side.

Next, I moved on to an elderly man who was hypoxic. There is roughly 21 per cent oxygen in the air we breathe, and most of the oxygen that crosses from our lungs into our blood isn't even used. For a healthy

---

* In medicine, 'angio' is used to describe a procedure involving a blood vessel, and 'plasty' comes from the Greek word meaning 'moulded' or 'formed'. In this case, 'coronary angioplasty' is a process whereby a catheter is passed through a peripheral artery and guided up into the coronary arteries to treat a blocked or diseased vessel.

person, even after the blood has been pumped around to all the other organs and has given up the oxygen they need for survival, there is still up to 80 per cent left over. This man was receiving 100 per cent oxygen and still his lungs weren't functioning well enough to pass sufficient amounts of it on to his blood. His family sat around him as he struggled, despite having been started on non-invasive ventilation as a temporary holding measure. For the family, he was their only priority, the centre of their room. For me, he was on my list to assess whether or not he stood to benefit from admission to intensive care.

We are taught that this sort of assessment is always done independently, and that it should never be tainted by the reality of capacity problems. The idea is to approach the problem in this order:

Question 1: What do they *need*?
Question 2: How can I facilitate it?

I believe entirely in this approach. The ability to make appropriate admission assessments is one of an intensivist's most important and valuable skills. The reality was that there were no beds available on the intensive-care unit itself, but the imperative was that I block it out; it was a distraction that was unfair to the patient in front of me.

The consultant came and we had a long conversation. We went through the history and the X-rays and we spoke to his family. It was decided that the patient would not benefit from escalation to intensive care. This meant that he would go to the ward, with the expectation that he was now in the final days of his life. I agreed it was the right decision for the patient, but I was also genuinely relieved that had been the decision – I don't know how we would have found space for him. I moved on, hoping all night that the next patient I was asked to see wouldn't need a bed, and hoping also that I was good enough not to let that detract from my assessment of their needs.

Focus: it is a requirement, even when you are standing in the resus department and it feels like somebody has asked you to make a difficult decision while standing still in the centre of Waterloo Station in the middle of the rush hour. People who work in acute care adapt to become good at not needing peace and quiet to make their decisions. I find that I am learning this and I can manage it, as long as I still have access to a pen.

I am a fan of writing things down, and that clearly won't come as a shock to you, but perhaps because I am young and of the 'next generation' of consultants, you might think I ought to be putting out bunting to celebrate our movement in medicine towards embracing 'paperless records'. Personally, though, I have never been fond of the online, pro-forma way of recording matters. Of course I see that it has some strengths, but in my experience there is little room for free text and thinking out loud.

Instead, I value the simple tool of a pen, and wonder how I could possibly focus without it. Usually when I have this thought, I am in the resus department or out on the general wards and I have seen a patient who has been referred because the parent team is worried the patient might need a higher level of care. I arrive, go through the patient's background and admission history, then work my way through the blood results, any radiology or other imaging that is available and the records of vital signs. I speak to the patient, if they are able to communicate, and then I examine them. Next,

I take out a pen from the top pocket of my scrubs and I start to put it all together.

Invariably somebody from the patient's team will approach me, less than ten seconds after the pen comes out, and enquire, 'So, what's the plan then?' I will look up from my page and tell them the same thing every time: 'I don't know; when I've finished writing, I'll have decided and I'll let you know.' That isn't me being rude, but there is so much to consider. What are the patient's problems? Which of them are a priority now? Do we have a treatment for them? Do they want it? Do we think they would benefit? What does 'benefit' mean anyway?

Usually, within a couple of minutes, somebody else will have approached and asked me the same question: 'So, what's the plan then?'

Don't misunderstand me – I don't advocate sitting down with your pen beside an acute asthmatic, haemorrhaging patient or someone in cardiac arrest, but many of the admission decisions I make are less urgent than that. It is possible to be both rational and thorough; I just need to cope with the environment that I find myself in and not get too distracted. I could be standing in a resus bay beside a man who may or may not have a reversible illness. His family are standing beside him, looking at me and waiting for me to tell them the plan. The nurse needs to know what to tell the bed manager; the referring doctors want to know the outcome of their referral; and around me, four other patients have their own problems and their own teams buzzing about them. I need to focus, so I raise my flag, which is the pen and a blank sheet of paper.

Every human on the planet has good days and worse ones. It is sobering to consider that how I feel on a particular day can have such a sizeable effect on a patient's journey – if I am distracted by things at home, grumpy and put out by a lack of cohesion within my team, or simply if I am tired. Tiredness is another unhelpful addition to the workplace. It is a distraction and, as far as distractions go, it is one that frustrates me the most, because I can't always focus my way out of it. There are occasions when tiredness makes me a different doctor.

The last time I remember using tiredness as an excuse it was 7 a.m. and I was just starting to congratulate myself on the end of another set of night shifts, when I got a call from the medical registrar telling me that an elderly patient had been moved from major injuries into the resus department; she was unconscious and barely breathing.

I hauled myself down the corridor and into the resus department, where I was met with a team of people who, like me, didn't know much about the woman before them. I took the plastic mask and inflatable bag from the trolley next to me and, while pressing the mask onto her face and pulling up the jaw with one hand, I started hand-ventilating the patient, squeezing the bag with the other hand. I asked if somebody could go and find the junior doctor who had clerked the patient when they arrived in the emergency department a few hours beforehand. I'd have read the notes myself, but both my hands were otherwise occupied, ventilating the patient. To be honest, I also found myself highly irritated by the fact that nobody seemed to be able to give me a coherent history, and so when the junior doctor arrived I was probably less kind to him than I would have liked.

Looking back, I wasn't overtly mean, but I was undoubtedly grumpy, irritable and tired. I think I forgot to tell him that he wasn't in trouble, this wasn't an inquisition; I just needed an overview, quickly, to help me make some decisions, quickly. Though in retrospect, I am sure it must have felt like an inquisition.

The junior doctor stuttered his way through the patient's history and his reasons for presenting to the emergency department that night. Having decided that the patient should indeed be escalated to intensive care, I started off by intubating her and putting her on the ventilator. Over the next half-hour, her blood pressure plummeted and she proved difficult to stabilise. Somewhere in the midst of all this, I was suddenly and inconveniently confronted with how tired I was. In situations like this, I could usually think two or three steps ahead of what I was doing, but now every thought was wading slowly through treacle towards me.

The patient remained unstable; somebody still needed to speak to her family, who were waiting anxiously for news, and somebody needed to put their mind to figuring out what had happened to cause her deterioration in the first place. I looked at this woman, who was on the verge of something final, and I felt weighed down by the thought that she deserved a brain as sharp as a razor. Mine felt about as lethal as a butter knife. I felt anything but agile. Sometimes, after a night shift, a doctor or nurse might tell you that they arrived home and didn't really remember having driven there. They drove that familiar route home on autopilot, not even aware until they were home that they were perhaps less than fully conscious. At the end of that night shift, I was not experienced enough to stabilise this patient on autopilot.

I looked up at the clock, which read 7.55 a.m., and decided there was no reason to keep going when I knew I wasn't at my best. So I picked up the phone, knowing that the consultant would have arrived for the morning handover. He came into resus, friendly, fresh and smiling. I just looked at him pathetically and said, 'I'm so tired.' As a doctor, I cannot tell you how hard it is to use those words as an excuse. Objectively, it makes no sense that that should be the case, but it is the truth about the sort of culture we are immersed in and the standards we have set for ourselves. Looking back on that morning, I can tell myself there are so many things to feel guilty about: that I had not tied that patient up in a more complete package in time for the morning team; that I hadn't been nicer to the junior doctor; that I was tired, and that tiredness had distracted me from being the best I could be. I can easily reply to myself, too, that I'd have felt worse if I'd harmed her; I'd have felt worse if my communication with the family wasn't up to scratch, or if I'd missed something. I know all these things are true, but I still feel disappointed that it happened.

Incidentally, when the day registrar arrived after the consultant, he swooped into the resus bay and gleefully announced to me that he had managed, on the first attempt, to put an arterial line in my patient. He knew that I had failed twice. I looked at him through tired eyes after my four long shifts as he made an audible celebratory 'Yes!' noise and punched the air. For all my disappointment that I had not been exactly who I wanted to be that morning, given the same choice, I'd still rather be me.

Distraction also comes to me in forms that are more benign, and arguably more helpful. When I buy a patient a newspaper, or when somebody takes their friend in hospital some chocolates and a trashy magazine, what is that but an attempt at ensuring there is some distraction available to them? Routinely, when a patient wakes up from major surgery, I make a point of telling them how well they've done and suggest that it must be a relief to have at least that part of their journey behind them. Then I say something positive like, 'At least you might sleep better tonight than last night.' Usually they smile, then agree and say it is a relief and that yes, they didn't sleep a wink the night before the 'big op'. Most of these patients have a longer road ahead of them: one of chemotherapy, radiotherapy or further surgeries; still, it seems fitting to encourage the shorter-sighted distraction that celebrates those small milestones.

That's not to say that I want my patients to see things through rose-tinted spectacles. When I meet patients in intensive care, they are at their most vulnerable. These patients are the ones who come back from theatre, alert and entirely lucid, for a period of high-dependency monitoring. Usually they will have a urinary catheter, multiple venous cannulas and another line in their artery, to provide constant blood-pressure monitoring. They find themselves unable to mobilise, tethered to the bed by monitoring, sometimes in a single room, but more frequently with strangers to the left and right of them; strangers who may be intubated and ventilated, or delirious; strangers who most likely make it near-impossible to forget the worst fears they have for themselves. So yes, for these patients I engage in distraction, because I think it is kind.

I believe there are times when consultants have done the same for me. I remember one day I was leaving work after a difficult day, which had been overshadowed by the tragic death of a new mother. If you've got this far in the book, you will already have realised that there is a lot of death in intensive care. Some deaths, however, acquire an extra layer of solemnity about them. They're the deaths when the unit becomes noticeably silent and, for a time, everyone connected to it moves slowly, as if the air around them has thickened. On this day a consultant stopped me and said, 'I want you to know you were wonderful today.' Was I wonderful? I'm not sure; it is more likely that I just did my job, but I think the point he was making was for me to remember exactly that: I did my job. When I got in my car and drove home, I could spend the journey contemplating the depths of seemingly random trag-edy burdened upon the people I meet, or I could ask myself if I did my job well that day. That consultant wanted me to think about the latter.

We are all familiar with mantras and wise words on how banishing distraction is the path to success. Dis-traction has a bad reputation, but if you came to work in intensive care, you might believe me when I say that sometimes it is distraction that holds us together. Distraction has the power to keep us from stagnating in moments that would otherwise overwhelm us.

We doctors have also evolved to use humour to distract ourselves from all sorts of things. We laugh at things that other people most certainly don't. As a registrar in intensive care, it is part of my job to super-vise the safe transport of patients who are unstable, or on ventilators and various infusions of drugs, around the hospital. One day as I sat in our evening meeting, where we hand over the care of patients to the incom-ing team, I picked up the phone to answer a page and was met with shouting from a neurosurgical registrar. He was shouting at me for not having taken a now-dead patient for a CT head-scan. The torrent of rage erupted from a colleague who had previously always called himself by a shortened version of his first name. Now he was 'Mr'.

In a raised voice he said, 'This is a disgrace, we need this man's scan – it's been hours!'

His comical rant went on, and twice I intervened to tell him that the patient had died, and then again to say that I couldn't take a dead patient for a scan. But he wasn't really listening. Eventually the message got through, and the neurosurgeon exclaimed in disbelief, 'But no! I thought he went to intensive care?'

'No,' I said with half a smile. 'That's what I've been trying to tell you. I promise you he went to the morgue.'

The patient in question had died, following a long and difficult resuscitation attempt on the ward. We did everything we could to keep him going, but we failed and he died, with more than one neurosurgical consultant and registrar in attendance. How this surgeon thought the patient was still waiting for me to take him for a CT head-scan, hours later, is a mystery.

I put down the phone and turned back to my group, to carry on discussing the two pages of critically unwell patients before us: the car crashes, the overdoses, the infections you wouldn't wish on your worst enemy. I would be lying if I said that the phone call hadn't caused some smiles around the table – actually, I would go so far as to say the surgeon's comic disbelief had most definitely cheered us all up. Not in a callous way. Not in a way that was intended to disrespect the man we could not save, or to undermine the hours we had spent trying to achieve a different outcome. Just in the way 'we do', I guess. People call it gallows humour – grim humour in a desperate or hopeless situation. It is a joke despite an unpleasant outcome: the man was in the morgue, and I couldn't take him for that CT scan of his head because we couldn't save him. It's a comment that makes you laugh in the face of something that's not funny; he was not even fifty years old, and he was lost to his family. Nobody could save him now: not this neurosurgeon, and not even the best neurosurgeon in the world.

Humour is just something that we do to get through the day, and I think it had to be okay, because the joke wasn't really about a patient. The joke was about death – that miserable, shapeless, constantly looming cloud that hangs around us. Humour is a private distraction and, really, can you blame us?

Distraction

On the night the young man who had hanged himself was brought in, I broke the bad news to the family and, when I had finished, I left the room to answer a page. The medical registrar wanted me to come to the emergency department to see an elderly lady with sepsis, who he thought might need some drugs to support her circulation. In intensive care, it is important to have a picture of what the patient's physiological reserve is, so I began enquiring about how physiologically fit she was.

'Can she mobilise?' I asked him.

'Yes, I mean she uses a walking frame, but she'll have a chat with you – she can have a joke.'

I laughed, and told him that I tended not to make admission decisions based on how funny a person was; and when I put down the phone, I laughed again out loud while picturing the idea of demanding that patients do a stand-up comedy routine before they are allowed into intensive care. It distracted me from the reality of what I had just done; from the face of the mother I had looked at and to whom I had said, 'I'm sorry, but your son is going to die.' Sometimes you need to latch onto that sort of distraction when it presents itself. Sometimes you have to make some things funny.

At other times it is a patient who delivers the gift of laughter to me. At the end of the night shift, it is usual for the medical juniors to do a morning ward-round, in order to see all the new patients who have been admitted during their shift with the on-call consultant. One morning, in the middle of one of these very long and hectic post-take ward-rounds, an elderly lady with dementia grabbed me by the arm in front of a very lovely and mild-mannered consultant. She dug her nails into my arm, peering at me through narrowed eyes, and said, 'I know what you've done, Missy, it's written all over your face!' This was followed quickly by 'I know you're pregnant.' Then, keeping hold of my arm, she raised her other hand up and pointed her bony finger straight at my consultant, before screaming, loud enough for the whole ward to hear: 'AND I KNOW IT'S YOUR BABY!' My consultant found that he suddenly had to go and retrieve something from the nurses' station and hurried out of the bay. I was flagging, already past the end of my twelve-and-a-half-hour shift, and I would return for another shift in less than eleven hours now. How could I not grab that moment and laugh?

Distraction is the part of my day that comes and goes in waves and I think, on balance, I have to be grateful for it. Even with many more years ahead of me than there are behind me, I have worked in intensive care long enough to be able to look around me and recognise that, without the right distraction, we are at risk of succumbing to the harsh reality of it all. It's crucial for doctors to let in the light while it's there; to allow ourselves some relief.

I started off this chapter by recalling a time when I stood beside a young man who died by suicide. Outside these encounters, I don't know if I have any right to talk about suicide. The truth is that it hasn't really affected my life as it has affected thousands of families across the country, and I have a reverence for those who cope with the aftermath. I have a respect that tells me not to put my own spin on somebody's else's tragedy; you can never really know the entire truth of what forced the hand of the person who took their own life.

Suicide has become a talked-about topic among doctors of my generation, although it is something that perhaps we should talk about more. Recently, when another junior doctor's suicide was reported by the media, I had a text message from my youngest sister: 'Promise me you'd never do that.' My sister's close friend died by suicide when she was a teenager. My sister had read in the newspaper about a junior doctor who worked hard and was said to love her job. She read about somebody who, for all the detail that was reported, could have been me, and so she needed me to say that I wouldn't do that. I promised her.

There was a time when I didn't have any faces to put to doctor suicides. But in the past year alone, I have had more than a few. I know the intensity of sadness that I feel when I see these faces is at least in part because empathy is amplified when you can directly relate to something. As a doctor, I feel the burden of knowing these doctors are me – but for the grace of *something*. One morning, I attended a trauma call for another patient who had tried to end his own life. The patient was conscious, but distressed. I tried to calm him down and keep him still, and it took a couple of minutes for anyone to recognise the patient as a doctor from another hospital. Standing over his head that morning, I felt panic like I had never felt beside a patient before. It wasn't because I knew him as a colleague; I didn't. I didn't know his name and he wasn't even that close to my age. I had never shared a single moment with this man, but now I knew that we shared this job and I felt despairingly unnerved.

He started to list all the things he did not want our team to do, as part of our attempts to stabilise his condition. He used the medical words, the names of procedures. He told me that, if it came to it, he wished not to be considered for cardiopulmonary resuscitation. He pleaded with me to go and get a form to document this. Standing at the head-end of the patient put me in a prime position to be the recipient of all of these fraught instructions. I recall desperately trying to find a way to subtly get the A&E consultant's attention and, when I did, the only thing I had to say was a rattled statement of fact: 'He is a doctor,' I mouthed. The A&E consultant looked at me kindly and replied, 'It's okay.'

It is okay. Yes, okay.

We carry on.

So I went back to the resuscitation attempt, back to the fixing and focusing.

The evidence will tell me that my profession does not, of course, hold a monopoly on the burden of mental-health problems. Still, there are times when I have to think: There, but for the grace of *what*, go I?

What does all of this unease point to? For a doctor, the ability to try and really understand every patient in terms of their own narrative is a vastly important skill, but it is not a benign burden to bear, and it is not a straightforward load to balance on top of your own fragile, imperfect shoulders. If you ask any intensive-care doctor of my generation what their single biggest fear for their career ahead is, I believe they will tell you it is burnout. Burnout is my biggest fear: the idea that one day all the intensity might finally become too much for me, that I will lose my energy, my ability to respond emotionally to a situation, or my reliable sense of immense engagement in what I do. Who would I be then? What would I call myself? As Alice asks herself in *Alice's Adventures in Wonderland*: What does a flame look like after the candle has blown out?

First, however, she waited for a few minutes to see if she was going to shrink any further: she felt a little nervous about this; 'for it might end, you know,' said Alice to herself, 'in my going out altogether, like a candle. I wonder what I should be like then?' And she tried to fancy what the flame of a candle is like after the candle is blown out, for she could not remember ever having seen such a thing.

I am not naïve enough to think that distraction is a robust answer to many problems, but there are days when I think that respect for the value of a decent distraction is as good a fuel for my flame as anything else.

Anger

'Now you are a lioness,' said Aslan. 'And now all Narnia
will be renewed.'

C. S. Lewis, *Prince Caspian*

THE EARLIEST MEMORY I have of anger is when I am
about seven years old and my brother is ten. My brother
is, from a medical point of view, one in a billion. He was
born with a condition that at that time didn't even have
a name; a nameless condition that, ironically, made him
anything but nameless to everyone else. My brother's
appearance is different from that of the majority of
people, and he doesn't really fit into any of the boxes you
might have subconsciously made to recognise or group
together people with visible disability. When I was still
very young, there wasn't really a significant emotional
impact associated with that, because ordinary is just

what you happen to know. When my youngest sister was about three years old, we realised that she thought that 'a brother' was somebody who uses a wheelchair. She started asking how that person's brother *could* be their brother, when they didn't even have a wheelchair at all.

It didn't take me long to realise that, outside the enclosure of my family, my brother wasn't ordinary to other people. People had an interest, as humans do, and in truth while I don't blame them for their interest, I think I have to hold them accountable for their actions; and so many people were less than kind. From the age of about seven, I steadily became aware of the people who stared and turned their heads round by almost 180 degrees as they walked past us. I don't know exactly how to describe that feeling I had as a child – the feeling of being aware every day that people of all ages were staring at a person whom you love and, more than anything, of just wanting them to stop. It was a hurt sort of sewn up inside anger.

I have sat feet away from people who have looked at my brother and whispered, made faces and laughed; from children who have stopped dead in the middle of a room, stood and shouted, 'Hey, look at him!' As a young teenager, I was approached by a grown man, who demanded that I take my brother home because he was 'scaring' *his* children. I stood up to that man and told him to leave my brother and me alone. I roared, and later I cried myself to sleep.

I remember that I would try and hunt the stares of passers-by; fix them with my eyes, in an effort to pounce on them before my brother or parents noticed. I remember being obsessive about it as I walked alongside him, trying to bat away all those faces. I don't know why I thought this was my responsibility. I am sure the stares were noticed anyway, but I made it my task and, for better or for worse, this is a large part of what made me the doctor I am today.

It was the first consultant I ever worked for who referred to me as a lioness, and it made me feel proud. Females in medicine often go through the indignity of raising their heads above the parapet, only to be referred to in veiled negative terms, such as 'feisty'. That isn't universal, but it still happens. It doesn't take a young doctor any time at all to recognise that, aside from all the good, there is still much injustice in our health service. There is still so much wrong that is worth making better.

I do get angry. It is absurd that I should be half-afraid to admit that. I don't remember ever taking an oath not to be angry, but amongst medical profession-als we are still taught to consider it very much a dirty word. Personally, I think a little anger can be a good thing. Anger is just a flag that tells us we don't agree with something; but the key to getting the best out of anger requires recognising that its value is mostly lost after that first split-second. The goal is to turn it into something else: passion, inspiration, motivation, instruction. I'm not saying that anger is a virtue, but I am saying you need to respect that fire inside you.

General David Hurley, former Chief of the Austra-lian Defence Force, has been credited with a phrase that is now widely used across the NHS: 'The standard you walk past is the standard that you accept.' Throughout my career I know I will be confronted by many things that I feel are less than acceptable. The daily level of exposure becomes so chronic at some point that to allow any sort of fire to burn inside you is an effort that needs to be supported. Having an appropriate amount of anger isn't optional; it is necessary and, as a doctor, you have to respect what anger is telling you and use it to stand for something. I know I would want my own doctor to stand for something. None of this is the primary reason I became a doctor; but it is certainly the case that I feel responsible for defending the needs of a great many more people now than when I was a child.

People like to ask doctors if they chose their career because they wanted 'to help people'. It's the party line: what you're expected to say, to which many doctors will probably roll their eyes in response. 'Helping people' sounds like a lofty ambition, but for the very vast majority of people, the reality of our jobs is not about large-scale change. Being a doctor is not about aiming to change the world, but about making a difference to one person's world for a moment, or a month, or whatever amount of time they happen to pass through your hands. If I had wanted the ability to change the world on a phenomenal level, I'd have gone into scientific research or become a politician.

But we do want to help people, or at least the people in front of us, which is no small responsibility. Doctors are, for the most part, enthusiastic, highly driven individuals, and our sheer will and determination to do our own job to the best of our ability – in a pressurised environment where the stakes are high – can make us less than kind to each other. We become hardened to learn from others' mistakes, to view all actions from the harsh perspective of retrospect. We can forget that the latest, seemingly unnecessary referral, even when it seems undoubtedly an inappropriate one, was unlikely to be a deliberate plan to sabotage your working day.

On one occasion I hadn't yet finished taking the morning handover of patients on the unit when I got an urgent message calling me to A&E immediately. The consultant said, 'You'd better run. I'll fill you in later.'

There are different ways to be summoned by a bleep. The least urgent is just a couple of bleeps with an extension number that flashes on the screen; in this case, you might decide to finish what you are doing before returning the call. In an emergency you are summoned with a different sort of noise and a crackly voice-message telling the relevant team where to go and when: 'Trauma team to A&E resus in ten minutes.'

The most urgent type of emergency is generally alerted to you by a couple of fast bleeps and a voice telling you, specifically, to go somewhere immediately. On this particular day it was: 'Intensive-care registrar to A&E resus immediately.'

I left and scurried down two flights of stairs, along a corridor, turned left in the foyer, down to the end of another corridor, left again, through some double doors. The coffee I had been drinking at handover slid slightly back up my throat as I continued through the major-injuries department before arriving to meet one patient, one advanced clinical nurse practitioner and one charge nurse in the resus department.

'Intensive-care registrar,' I said, panting. 'You called me?'

The nurse practitioner started off his tale at a seemingly leisurely pace, telling me about the history of the presenting complaint. Catching my breath, after half a minute or so, I stopped him: 'Can you just tell me the emergency bit, and we'll get to all that afterwards?'

'What?'

'The emergency bit that you called me for. You know: A, B, C or D?'

A, B, C and D are the four pillars of emergency re-suscitation:

Airway
Breathing
Circulation
Disability/Neurological

When you get to 'E', it stands for 'everything else'.

'Oh, well, we haven't got intravenous access and we've estimated probably 500ml of blood loss,' he responded.

The provision of 'access' – intravenous or otherwise – comes under C for 'circulation', and is important as a precursor to replacing lost circulatory volume, as well as for giving drugs. I looked at the monitor: the heart rate beeped along at a profoundly normal 72 beats per minute, mean arterial blood pressure was normal, oxygen saturations were 100 per cent, with a normal respiratory rate. I looked at the patient: she was awake and alert. Granted she had pale lips and a pressure dressing on her groin, but no active bleeding.

'Has anyone else here in the department tried to establish access?' I asked in disbelief and irritation.

'No.'

'Have you looked for a vein with the ultrasound?' I continued, for no other reason than wanting to hear him say no.

'No,' he replied.

'And that's what you put out the fast bleep for?'

The practitioner now seemed irritated. 'Yes. Do you think it was inappropriate to call you?'

'No,' I answered, trying to level my tone. 'You're always welcome to ask for help, but I think it was an inappropriate use of an emergency fast bleep. Anyway, let's leave that for later.' I said it in a tone that did not match my fake pretence of not being annoyed. I definitely thought it was inappropriate.

The charge nurse wheeled the ultrasound into the cubicle and I placed two cannulas into the patient's arm. The practitioner had gone to the bench to write his notes and, feeling my usual remorse for being uncivil, I approached him and said I was sorry if I had seemed grumpy, but I really didn't feel it was an appropriately triaged call. I explained that I had left a handover and had literally run to help him. I didn't want to start changing my behaviour because I'd begun to doubt if something was an emergency at all.

The patient was still stable, so I left, a slave to that little black-boxed relic of one-way communication, knowing that I would always run, without questioning it.

I am, of course, aware that my anger isn't always seen as reasonable. If it is the tail end of the sugar-crash that comes routinely after a long week of night shifts, I can be a bit territorial when it comes to my patients.

At 6 a.m. on my fourth consecutive night shift, a prison guard was chained to a patient. He was standing behind the head of the bed, straight-backed and with his feet spread apart, with a long metal chain draped between him and the patient's wrist. A second guard sat on a chair in the corner of the room. The patient himself, a male in his forties, lay in bed, intubated, sedated and, to the best of my knowledge, unaware of the world around him.

'Why are you chained to him?' I opened with this line when I entered the room, quickly adding, 'You can't stand there, anyway.'

I looked at the guard who stood behind the bed. I was annoyed, but was going for a tone that conveyed disbelief. The prison guard returned a stare as firm as my own and said that he would continue to be chained to the patient until the governor said otherwise.

'Well, you can't stand *there*, that's my spot.'

The truth was that I didn't actually need to stand there at all. I mean, I might at some stage. If there was an emergency, that *was* my spot, and the nurse had already moved the guard away from the space around her writing station.

'Anyway,' I continued, 'there really is no reason for you to be chained to him – he literally can't even breathe.'

The guards looked back at me as if I had naïvety oozing out of my eyeballs. 'He's Category A,' I was told.

Category A?

'Well, he's category ventilated and sedated now, and if something happens and I need to shock him, don't be surprised if you get electrocuted, because I have already told you that I don't want you to be chained to him.'

I was tired and I was being unreasonable, but that was *my* patient. The chances of me actually having to deliver a shock to this patient for cardiac arrhythmia were about as high as the chances of these two prison guards obeying my every command. But we had admitted this patient to hospital and, for the moment, had taken away his mental capacity, by putting him in this situation. Now it was my responsibility to protect him.

In *The Lion, the Witch and the Wardrobe* the lion Aslan roared and C. S. Lewis proclaimed, 'Wrong will be right, when Aslan comes in sight, At the sound of his roar, sorrows will be no more.' In a busy hospital, things aren't really that simple, and many of my own roars are entirely ineffective. This patient was a critically unwell man, and I wanted to give out some sort of critical-illness amnesty, at least while he couldn't even breathe for himself.

The guards looked back at me, unemotional, with faces that said, 'Governor says no.'

What crime had that man committed? Something terrible, maybe. Did I care? Honestly, not at all.

We are taught to adopt this attitude of neutrality. This man was my patient and I wanted to treat him like anybody else. Medicine just doesn't work, otherwise – we cannot invent a moral hierarchy within the walls of intensive care. I was angry on my patient's behalf, but from one perspective some people might see me as presiding over a prison of a different sort. After all, none of the patients surrounding me were truly free to leave. Intensive care is an alien place. Patients like this man lie in beds with a tube in their throat, in a drug-induced state of coma. They have a tube for urine to come out, and a tube for food to go in. For that time they have no voice, no capacity to choose their interaction with the world.

The environment of intensive care nips away at what it is to be human and, if you're not careful, patients can become dehumanised. They become organ systems, they become numbers. So, as a doctor, you have to make priorities for yourself; you have to have the strength to clutch consistently at the dignity that you think you can preserve, and call it sacred.

There is a consultant who frequently tells me that nobody comes to work to do a bad job. That line in itself probably doesn't seem particularly profound, but if you find yourself enraged amidst memories of your own actions, or the actions of others, then accepting that nobody in the room is *trying* to do a bad job is a powerful tool that can give you the headspace to figure out what the frame for the actions was in the first place. I think, when it comes to the medicalisation of death specifically, that the glare of public and legal scrutiny has some responsibility to bear. As healthcare professionals, there are times when the resulting realities of our practice make all of us angry.

There are times when I make my way to an emergency call on the wards and I know I am already walking alongside the Grim Reaper. I wonder if it hurts him to see the deathbeds we make for some people. I wonder if, as he walks the corridors beside me, it sometimes makes him angry, too. It is usually in the early hours of the morning, when the crackly voice from my bleep summons me. I will run-walk and arrive to stand at the end of the bed, like some sort of ghoulish arbitrator. Often it seems as though I'm supposed to give some sort of pseudo-permission: *'You may allow them to die now.'* It is an odd thing to consider this as part of your day-to-day life. The reality of many of these situations, of course, is that the Grim Reaper has already arrived and the circus of resuscitation is an illusion – an act that might make it appear as if we have some sort of control.

It was again 6 a.m. and I was standing at the end of another bed. Compressions had been stopped and the patient heaved what would be her final minutes of disorganised, agonal breaths. Her circulation was adrenaline-dependent and failing, and her pulse was barely palpable in the clammy creases of her groin. I had already spoken with my consultant and had advised the team that we felt further escalation to intensive care would not be appropriate. I could have walked away then, because I had done what they had called me there to do, but I didn't, because that's not the doctor I would want at the foot of my bed. And besides, I was not the only one who knew that the situation was unsalvageable. I am sure I wasn't the only one on the team who would rather not have put hands on the patient that night. So, we continue to work together.

I focused on what I thought I could do, which was to try and make her look as if she was about to die peacefully in her bed. I helped the night sisters lift the patient gently back up from where she had crumpled down into the middle of the mattress. I asked one of the other junior doctors to retrieve the pillow, from where it had been thrown aside on a chair. I wiped the patient's mouth. I put my hand on her forehead for a couple of seconds, and I don't know what that was supposed to mean, but I often feel obliged to do it. I think it makes me feel like I am paying some respect. Maybe it is an apology.

I looked at the other three bed spaces in that room, their paper curtains pulled round in a futile attempt to buffer those patients from what had unfolded just feet away from where they slept. I doubted any of them were sleeping. Then, turning to leave, I realised the medical registrar and his junior were preparing to get a venous blood sample from her groin.

Blood tests can tell you a lot about a patient's physiology. They might have told us some things here, but they would not have told us anything that would have helped that patient in her final minutes. In medicine, the burden of any treatment or procedure that we expose a patient to needs to be weighed against the benefit for that particular patient. The burden of that needle simply could not be held as necessary for that dying patient. I knew I was partially responsible for this predicament.

Anger

When I had arrived at the tail-end of the resuscitation attempt, it already felt abundantly clear that we weren't going to be 'successful'. One of the more junior doctors was desperately trying to get some blood samples from the patient's shut-down, cold peripheries, but the team had already secured a cannula for venous access and a couple of millilitres of blood for a blood-gas sample. That would provide enough information, so I told the junior to stop, nicely.

I didn't know the medical registrar who was leading the team that night, as he had joined to do a locum night shift and so was new to us all, but I looked at the night sister, who also appeared perturbed. And so I suggested, coolly, that taking further bloods wasn't necessary.

'We haven't got any,' was his answer.

'She is dying,' I replied. 'It won't change her management now, and you don't need it.'

'But she isn't dead yet – maybe we should still get one?'

It felt like a genuine question, but as the conversation continued, I moved from calm enquiry to direction, and finally to anger and exasperation.

'It is up to you, but this is not what I would want for my grandmother. Is it what you would want for yours?'

I am sure I raised my voice. There was silence. He didn't answer me, but he stopped and I walked away.

I cannot over-stress to you the cumulative burden of watching people spend their last moments in ways that you would not wish for anybody you loved. It is enough to make you defensive; it is enough to make you angry. It is enough to make you employ cynicism as a defence. One day it led me to feel anger towards a colleague who turned out to be the kindest person I had met that day.

It was already late into Saturday afternoon; hospital admissions were pouring in, and both the wards and the emergency department were struggling, backing up with all the discharges they couldn't sort out over the weekend. The air ambulance had called ahead about a man in his early seventies who had been found on the pavement in cardiac arrest.

Our patient arrived, packaged on a stretcher; intubated and ventilated. His heart had restarted in the ambulance, but still he struggled to maintain his own circulation. Shortly after arrival he had another cardiac arrest, so we started CPR again and eventually his heart began to beat once more. Over the next hour or so we managed his blood pressure and supervised his ventilation. We narrowly avoided two further cardiac arrests. When he was finally stable enough, we transported him for a CT scan of his head, thorax, abdomen and pelvis, but once the first images of his brain and cervical-spine injuries appeared, it was immediately evident that he would not survive.

He had come to us an unknown male. The police were unable to trace any of his relatives, and his pockets contained only a jumble of keys and coins and a receipt for milk. We put everything in a plastic bag, with the grey trousers and dark-green jumper that we had cut off his body, and his watch. There was no phone, no wallet, just this dying man without a name. While he was still intubated and on the ventilator, the emergency-department doctor and I set about trying to find a place for him to die. Dying was inevitable, and a bustling resus is no place to pass your final minutes, if it can be helped. This anonymous man lay on a trolley between the junction of two sets of open doors, and the curtains barely reached around the cubicle. The emergency-department doctor tried to reserve a side-room in the main department, but there were none to spare. 'Best try to get him to the acute medical ward,' we were told. My colleague phoned the patient-flow manager and begged for an urgent side-room. Against the odds for a Saturday afternoon, they had one – my heart lifted. But, the flow manager told us, they would not be able to take him just yet.

I grumbled angrily to myself about the flow manager. As we waited, my annoyance escalated to anger and then to despair, as I sat, feeling generally helpless, watching my patient and still hoping we could somehow find him a more comfortable place to pass his final moments, before it was too late.

After a relatively short time, the flow manager arrived in the resus department. She was a nurse and arrived in a hurry, expressing how sorry she was about the delay and explaining that she had wanted to make sure she found a member of staff who was free to be with the patient while he died. She had brought with her a healthcare attendant for that purpose, and a bed. She asked if I would wait to extubate him until he was cleaned up properly and had been transferred off the hard trolley. Then she wheeled him away to the room, and my anger dissolved into gratitude. When I walked past later, I saw that she had left him not only a hand to hold, but her phone beside him on the pillow, playing Mozart.

The anger I feel in these situations is just that: anger at a situation. I try and remember the line that nobody comes to work to do a bad job, and that managing end-of-life issues while taking into account the growing legal framework – within the time and resource constraints of an acute hospital setting – is genuinely difficult. And also, that I'm not the only one who cares.

Words are so important. I can use words within a context that seem perfectly reasonable to me, but words in a conversation usually only mean whatever the person you are speaking to thinks they mean. There was a time in my first year as a doctor when I sat down to explain to a family that their elderly relative was dying. I told them that we would focus now on controlling her symptoms as she died, and that we were going to start her on a care pathway that prioritised things that would help patients who were in their last days of life. I reached the end of the conversation and left the family with their relative, before returning about twenty minutes later to check how my patient was.

'Have you started the process?' was the question from her son.

'The process?' I was bemused, but trying not to show it.

'Yes,' he replied. 'I mean now she's on the pathway, have you started the dying process?'

Imagine my horror as I realised that her son thought I was to have some active role in inducing the death of his mother.

I had said nothing of the sort. Well, to my mind, I had said nothing of the sort. I sat down and started the conversation again. Now I don't ever say the word 'pathway' – not when it comes to dying; it just has the wrong connotations.

Often the things that make me angry at work are words: 'wheelchair-bound', 'poor historian' and 'demented' are the kind of phrases that can really get my back up. If you say those words in my presence, you will see my lip curl – I can't hide it, even though I know it has often led to glances of irritation. I know it can foster dislike and, honestly, sometimes I look back and feel the same about myself.

Once, I was looking after a patient who had transitioned from care that was intended to get him home, to care that would support him in his last days of life: 'care of the dying', as it is called. At evening handover, it came to my attention that the handover document, which was regularly updated by one of the more junior doctors, had described this plan as 'withdrawal of care'.

Instinctively, I could not ignore that. 'Pick some other words, and take that off the handover,' I immediately interjected.

My more junior colleagues looked up from their sheets of paper, and one replied indifferently, 'What do you want us to say?'

The answer was anything that didn't suggest that we stopped caring for somebody who was dying. There was also the follow-up question: 'Why can't we say that anyway?' They had a point. For my colleagues, the words wouldn't really change the care given to our patient, and I knew that; but the words were still important. And you might wonder why, in the context of a job looking after critically unwell patients, I should bother to sweat this small stuff anyway?

Sweating the small stuff is a bit of an unfashionable thing to do these days. When you call something small, I think there is suddenly pressure to just let it go. I've often thought this is an unfair connotation to tie to the word 'small'; we're told to appreciate the 'little things', but not to sweat the 'small stuff'. When should the size of something generate wonder and gratitude, and when should it be brushed off entirely?

One of the things I try to remember about being a doctor is that every meeting I have with a patient will almost invariably be more significant to them than it is to me. This means I have to accept that I am a bad judge of what the 'small stuff' actually is. It seems, on this basis, such an easy answer to aim to choose all your words with other people's feelings in mind. I have been that member of the public who has been hurt by the words of a doctor. I have seethed with anger at a junior doctor who decided to scrawl carelessly, 'Wheelchair, spina bifida' in the indications box of an X-ray request for my brother, as if a wheelchair was somehow an indication for an X-ray, and with sheer abandonment of the fact that my brother doesn't even have spina bifida. He would still get his X-ray, and it would be the same X-ray, irrespective of the words the doctor had chosen to write on that little yellow card; but as the relative of a patient, that sort of absent-minded carelessness mattered hugely to me. So I sweat the small stuff. I consider how every word I say might make a patient feel.

One night I was called to see Greg, a middle-aged man with recurrent and now metastatic pancreatic cancer. The medical registrar had picked up the phone to call me at about midnight, and she explained that Greg had sepsis and had reached the point where normally we would have to consider blood-pressure support. She explained to me that there was nothing in the notes to signal what sort of thoughts his team or the patient had on immediate management priorities. It was inconvenient for me that the oncology team, who knew him, hadn't already broached the topic of resuscitation or escalation to intensive care during daylight hours, but when I looked on the computer system, I saw that the last clinic letter recorded that they had only recently broken the very poor prognosis to him. They wrote at the time that he was 'devastated', and I presume that was quite enough for one day, so I understood.

I told the medical registrar I was on my way, but also asked if she could call oncology at home anyway and discuss where they saw Greg's care progressing. I arrived on the ward while the medical registrar was still on the phone, and I began to look through his notes. At the end of the initial medical admission notes from the day before, I spotted a single line of writing: 'Would like to be resuscitated and artificially ventilated, if required.'

I understood that care planning had not quite caught up with the progression of Greg's illness, but I found it so much harder to be understanding about that line in his notes: 'Would like to be resuscitated and artificially ventilated, if required.'

Required for what? There was no context. Required for life, perhaps? Had we offered this man a chance at life?

In Harry Potter's world, there is something called the Mirror of Erised. Erised is 'desire' spelt backwards, and the idea is that you stand in front of the mirror and see what is the most desperate desire of your heart. You see yourself living that dream. I don't think you need be the most intuitive person to guess what Greg would see, if he stood in front of that mirror.

The stark, inflexible truth was that he *was* going to die, and soon. Of course end-of-life matters needed to be discussed; but had we asked him if he wanted to live, or had we asked him how he wanted to die?

I went to see the patient. He was dressed in shorts and a dark-green T-shirt and lay on top of a made bed. He lay there with a body that looked far too reliable to be that ill, and a face that looked disappointed, detached even, from everything that surrounded him. When I returned to the nurses' station, the medical registrar had finished her conversation with oncology. She told me that the team didn't feel intensive care was an appropriate option and they would discuss this with their patient, so I left.

Situations like this make me sceptical about the legislation that surrounds some potentially life-saving treatments, like CPR. I often wonder whether any of it has had the desired effect of making us better at discussing and dealing with important end-of-life issues, or simply fearful of appearing to stay on the right side of the law. When a patient comes into A&E dying from complications of metastatic pancreatic cancer, and we feel obliged there and then to follow a protocol and formally address the issue of escalation and limitation of treatment options, do we ask the right questions?

Do you want to live? Or: *How do you want to die?*

It's just not the same thing.

I have had what I am sure is an average number of run-ins with angry patients. Sometimes this anger comes from a recognised pathology, like the twenty-year-old who had been in a road-traffic accident and sustained some contusions to his lungs and multiple rib fractures. His rib injuries meant it was difficult for him to breathe, and the contusions to his lungs meant that large parts of his lungs were less capable of facilitating the transfer of oxygen into his blood. As a result he was hypoxic and, when your brain is deprived of oxygen, it can make you an angry person. He told me that if I even thought about 'putting him to sleep', he would find and 'fucking kill' me. Obviously, because he did not have mental capacity and it was undoubtedly in his best interests, I did put him to sleep and I placed him on a ventilator. He woke up a few days later, improved and, to the best of my knowledge, without any impulse to plan my murder.

Intensive care is a hotbed for delirium. You can be the most mild-mannered, upstanding gentleman in the world, but when the alien surroundings of intensive care meet your deranged physiology, you might find yourself throwing your water jug across the room at a nurse. More than once I have crawled on my hands and knees around the back of a bed in intensive care to co-vertly inject an anti-psychotic through the central line of a shouting, angry and delirious patient, just to keep them from causing themselves very serious harm.

I have been spat at by an elderly lady with dementia, who was convinced I was stopping her from catching a bus home; punched in the arm by a man who was fright-ened and had no idea why there was a catheter in his bladder. I have been smacked in the legs by a patient's walking frame. This sort of anger is blameless and, at times, even comical in its presentation, but it is equally important to remember that a lot of the anger we see, even where a patient has a condition like dementia, is an attempt at communicating a need for something.

I learned that from Jack. Jack carried his memories in a small brown leather photo album under his arm, by his bedside or in his pocket. He had dementia and was no longer able to live in his own home. He initially came to us because he had flu, but ended up staying on for a few weeks after his recovery, while appropriate care in the community was arranged.

Jack ran on his own time and, as one of those patients who sat somewhere in the gap of not being strictly 'ill', but still not having a suitable place to go, we tried to be accommodating. So we got used to his preference for sleeping in a little, and we would allow breakfast to wait. Jack became a fixture on the ward, and I liked his company. When he spoke, there was a light behind his eyes that made me expect to hear a riddle or a joke. He reminded me of my own grandad, and when there was a quiet moment I tried to sit beside him and ask about the photographs in his book.

One day when I was sitting at the nursing station writing notes, Jack walked over with a plastic beaker in his hand. Bang, bang, bang! He began to hit the counter with the beaker repeatedly, and the noise echoed boisterously through the long ward of patients.

'Could you stop that, please, Jack?' I asked, looking up from my work. He said no. Actually he said something much less polite than 'no', and then told me exactly what I should do with myself.

Bang, bang, bang! The noise continued, even louder, as Jack bashed that beaker onto the surface of the desk with all his might. I asked if maybe he'd like to go for a walk with me. Again, the negative, the expletive; and the banging just grew louder and louder.

A colleague who was working at the desk beside me turned round on her chair and calmly and quietly enquired, '*Why* are you making that noise, Jack?'

The banging stopped.

Jack paused, before replying earnestly, 'I'm sending out distress signals to the ships.'

'Oh, really?' she replied. 'And do you think our little hospital is equipped to handle all these ships, when they arrive?'

'I don't know,' Jack replied, and he smiled and stopped. Then she offered him a chair. Jack put down the beaker, and they continued a conversation while she typed away beside him at a discharge letter. Fifteen minutes later they were still talking, and had moved the conversation on to what it was like to be an economic migrant to England in the 1950s.

Jack's anger was really a justifiable need for something. And even in the absence of neurological disease, the patients and relatives I meet often find themselves in situations where they use anger to disguise emotions that are much more complicated. Medicine would be so easy, if patients and doctors started every conversation with a real understanding of where the other person was coming from, but real practice isn't like that. We have to do our best to figure each other out as we go along.

It was almost the end of one of those days that had gone quite well. It had been relatively quiet, without being tiresome. The sort of day where you can sneak off in the evening and get yourself a hot chocolate from the coffee shop. I was paying for this, when my bleep went off. I took the referral and, before I put down the phone, the referring doctor added a hasty footnote: 'Just a warning for when you get here: his wife is a very angry woman.'

I sighed, but at least I had got the hot chocolate. When I arrived, the surgical registrar rehashed the patient's history of diabetes, multiple diabetic foot-ulcers and high blood pressure. Now he needed his leg amputated and, owing to resulting sepsis, it was urgent. But the patient was refusing surgery. It was expected that if he did have surgery, he would be significantly unwell post-operatively, and so the team asked if we would support the patient in intensive care after surgery.

Knocking back the last of my hot chocolate, I noticed a junior doctor on the ward looking pleased with himself, as if he knew he was about to get some quality entertainment. 'Are you going in to see them?' he asked, eyebrow raised and shifting his head in the direction of the bay of patients. Then he gave me a smile that said: 'I'm going to wait here, so I can see your face when you come out.' It seemed that every member of staff had had a run-in with the angry wife.

'Right,' I said resolutely. 'Well, I'm going to go into that room and do everything in my power not to be offended.'

The man, who introduced himself as David, was in his seventies and lay propped up on two pillows in bed. His wife sat with a sour expression in the padded seat next to the bed, facing the same direction as her husband, because there was no room in the little bed space to turn the chair another way. I pulled the curtains around their space and slid into the narrow gap between the bed and the window. I introduced myself to each of them in turn and then started with some 'break the ice' talk. I felt grateful I didn't have any particular pressure that day to be anywhere else. David explained to me that his wife was his carer. He went through his general history and symptoms in the weeks leading up to this admission, and then I directed the conversation towards the proposed plan for amputation and whether an admission to intensive care, post-operatively, would be acceptable to him. He reiterated that he would not consent to the surgery in the first place.

I don't know if this will be a surprise to you, but I have to admit that, as much as blood and guts don't bother me, there is something psychologically harrowing about the idea of one of my limbs being removed and sitting in a medical waste bin. Understandably, this is enormously difficult for any person to get their head around; and, understandably, it was difficult for David

Anger

to give less weight to the idea that sacrificing his limb was felt to be a life-saving measure, and more to focusing on the longer-term issue of how he would cope, in reality, with one leg.

His wife rolled her eyes a lot. I tried to give her a positive amount of eye contact, while still allowing the bulk of my focus to rest on David. She tutted at me when I spoke, and eventually interjected to tell me about all the careless things doctors had ever done. She told me quite clearly that, as far as she was concerned, we were all the same – and none of us could do our jobs correctly. I listened and reminded myself that I was not going to be offended. This was not the time to take the bait.

So my initial assessment confirmed that, yes, she was undoubtedly very angry. David, on the other hand, seemed mostly confused.

I moved on to examine him, and he continued to talk in a rather disorganised way about hoists and care, and how their son lived too far away now to help out at home. I'd almost lost the train of conversation completely, when I caught the end of a sentence that made me stop: '... and she's not going to be here anyway, are you?'

'Yes,' his wife replied tartly. 'I'm only here until I'm dead.'

I stopped and looked up at his wife, before enquiring tentatively what she meant. The answer came in the same tone of disdain and mistrust. Put simply, she had a terminal cancer diagnosis and her prognosis was less than a year.

I looked at that angry woman and felt my next breath fill up my insides with the enormity and sadness of what this couple had to face. I stood not just with a patient who was facing a decision that would permanently change how he existed in the world, but with a couple who were losing each other; and with a woman who was dealing with her own illness, while seething with the knowledge that she would be forced to leave her husband alone.

When I entered the room, I was both defensive and frightened of that woman's anger, but when I left, I did not fear her behaviour at all. I could not even condemn it.

Within the context of necessity and submission to the right sort of governance, perhaps it is true that 'Anger in its time and place, May assume a kind of grace,' as Charles Lamb writes in his poem 'Anger'. If I have any advice to give those who will enter this profession after me, I think it might be that they should retain the energy to roar, just a little, sometimes.

Disgust

Evermore in the world is this marvellous balance of beauty and disgust, magnificence and rats.

Ralph Waldo Emerson

IN THE GENERAL SENSE, I probably don't notice any more a lot of what you might think would disgust me. I have learned in practice to cope with most smells and sensations. I have got used to the fact that if a patient haemorrhages enough, their blood will clot, like deep-red glistening jelly, where it falls and will start to smell like meat from the butcher's. When I stood with my hands on a man who had been shot through the head, blood poured from his wounds. It seeped through the gauze that I had pressed there, rolled through the gaps in my fingers, down past the cuff of my gloves and dripped steadily onto my leg. I could feel the warmth of that blood as it seeped through the material of my scrubs. I lowered my forearms down either side of his head to keep him still, and the blood smeared itself across my bare skin. The team leader asked me to lift up the back of the patient's head and, as I did so, the pool of already congealed blood beneath it fell away. It slid and then splattered, right onto the canvas of my shoes.

The smell of blood takes me back to being fifteen years old, standing in a lab coat in front of a pig's heart in biology class, with a scalpel in hand and the girl next to me groaning, because she didn't even like to cut up raw chicken breast. The air in that memory is sticky with the same smell. The smell of something raw. At school, we had to supply the animal organs for dissection in biology class. My mam would order them from the butcher's and I'd carry body parts to school in plastic bags. Once, I left a cow's eyeball at home in the kitchen, so my mam dropped it off at school for me later. When I went at lunchtime to collect it from the reception desk, the secretaries sat noticeable feet away from the eyeball, where it rested on the counter in the same sort of transparent bag you might buy your minced beef in. They all looked thoroughly disgusted and gestured wildly for me to get it out of there, now.

I can wrestle with the stench of inspecting the bed-pan of black faeces, so that I can be sure it is really melaena that has occurred. The difference between just very dark-coloured stool and melaena, which is the result of haemorrhage from the upper digestive tract into the colon – aside from the unmistakable smell – is that if it is melaena, it should also be sticky, like tar.

The gurgle of custard-coloured sputum bubbling its way slowly out of a tracheal tube on deep suctioning can be oddly satisfying; and I can rise above the unpalatable process of lifting the lid of a sputum pot, to try and gauge whether or not a patient with bronchiectasis needs antibiotics. The trick to dealing with smells is to breathe through your mouth. This is counter-intuitive, because when faced with the stench of *Clostridium difficile* diarrhoea, the last thing you want to do is open your mouth and risk tasting it. I would also warn that this tip isn't recommended when you're undressing, for example, some chronic leg ulcers. Those bandages unravel and although the stench grows steadily, you must prepare for that final layer, which, when it unravels, creates a blizzard of tiny white flakes of skin and debris. I have learned the hard way when it's not advisable to breathe through your mouth.

Places we put our fingers. Memories of being wrist-deep in a manual evacuation of faeces. Stories of blood, pus, sputum and odour. These are all the stereotypically gruesome anecdotes. Really, however, they are the sort of experiences that I have just got used to and, entertaining as they may be, they are paltry in comparison to the things that can still really turn my stomach.

Think about the noise of hearing somebody's sternum break. The snap of bones. The hollow crunch of ribs that crack beneath your hands as you deliver CPR. The tension of a thorax that gives way to the heel of your hand when you push, push, push. 'Good compressions,' the automated voice from the defibrillator will call, and that voice is universally encouraging because it does not know whose body you are insulting. Then you stop, and somebody feels for a pulse – they've got one.

But now you leave the patient to die again, because the decision is that he would never survive to benefit from escalation to intensive care. That would have been true even before the CPR started.

'What is his name?' asks another doctor, and you answer that you don't actually know it. You look down at the wristband. You ask for a pillow, and the nurse tells you that they don't keep any pillows in A&E. She finds a blanket and rolls it up under his head.

I could tell that story several ways, but you will know by now that it is the story of many people. I could paint it rosier, add more details, but when I relive these cases, I often don't do so. Sometimes I choose to recall them just like that. Because I am so disgusted with myself, I recall the crack of that person's bones beneath my hands, and I remind myself of the feeling of knowing that person is already dead. I recall knowing that I am not helping.

The inharmonious indrawing of a broken sternum when a patient heaves their last breaths might not in itself make you feel nauseated, but imagine that you had caused this situation. Imagine they were *your* hands that had felt forced to carry out this task, and now you are watching while this human appears to suffer, for what will be their last seconds or minutes. You ought to feel nauseated at that. It's this kind of situation that makes me feel some empathy for Shakespeare's Macbeth when he cries, 'Will all great Neptune's ocean wash this blood clean from my hand? No, this my hand will rather the multitudinous seas incarnadine, making the green one red.' I wonder if I took to looking at my hands mournfully on these occasions, and actually reciting quotes of Shakespearian levels of tragedy, it might affect some change. It is probably more likely that I'd be told to slap myself and would be placed on some sort of stress-leave.

Even after many years now, there still remains for me something disgusting about the smell of the morgue: the smell of formalin. Formalin is a solution of formaldehyde in water, which is used as the basis for preserving corpses, or any other biological specimen really. I can't easily describe it to you, but the smell is unmistakable; and I can recall it, actively, at any given moment, if I choose to. It is easier if I am eating meat, and particularly, for some reason, if I am eating a ham sandwich. I remember that I am eating flesh and I recall the smell of the morgue and it is enough to put me off my lunch, or at least switch to something vegetarian. It isn't a fear of death or corpses that turns my stomach. It is the seemingly unearthly mixture of cold flesh that smells like formalin and the sheer enormity of death inside that room.

Usually when I visit the morgue, it is to check and release a body for cremation. I ring the bell. A voice answers from the intercom and I say something generic in response, like 'Crem viewing', before the door unlocks and I am let in. I declare the name of the patient I have an interest in, as I stand looking up at the long panel of fridge drawers, each marked with the name of a different patient. There are babies and children here, too; for those who did not live much life at all, the sign will just read 'Baby' and the family name: Baby Smith, Baby Brown, Baby Shah. I will see names of patients I have looked after or known, and every so often I will read the name of somebody I know has been in those fridges for far longer than average, because they are without a family to come and arrange a funeral.

The drawers run four high and about ten across. The arrangement makes up a wall of bodies and, when the chosen one is pulled out for me to inspect, I will sometimes have to climb a portable metal staircase to whichever level is required. From the staircase, it is possible for me to turn my head left or right, peer inwards and look down the line inside, to appreciate all those bodies stacked there in the icy air with their yellowed skin, sunken eyes and identical white hospital shrouds. I place my hand on the chest of the patient to do the obligatory and yet largely defunct 'pacemaker check'. When a body is released for cremation, I am one of two doctors who will sign a form to say, amongst other things, that I have examined the body and noted any metal that has the potential to cause an explosion. Pacemakers and internal defibrillators can explode during the process of cremation, so it is important that they are removed, but this act of checking is fairly pointless because I have never had a patient for whom I didn't already have a chest X-ray or some other imaging that would tell me if the patient had such a device; and because we are lucky to work with mortuary technicians who check that, too.

The disposable white shrouds that we use to clothe deceased patients in have a ruched neckline that reminds me of a choirboy's dress. It has often seemed to me like an incongruous and curious attempt, within the context of medicine, to keep something that is as regular as death in a hospital tied to something celestial and divine.

When it comes to the mortuary, there isn't a comfortable place inside my head that easily accommodates the spectacle of body stacked upon body – bunkbeds for corpses.

Feeling disgust as a reflex when the putrid pus of an appendicular abscess is released into the air of the operating theatre is one thing, but being disgusted by your patient is quite another.

I like to believe that, if one truly has respect for the complexity of the human condition, it isn't possible to feel pure, unadulterated disgust towards another person indefinitely. Life seems to me far too complex for unbridled disgust, but we all have our own moral standards and our own framework for judging other people's choices in life. Or, more accurately, to decide what we consider is a 'choice', as opposed to the product of a situation that is thrust upon someone. I am no different in this respect.

I can recall the things that have tested me. I have told you of my frustration with the word 'fighter' when applied to a patient's journey through any illness. It is not so much the connotations associated with having to be strong and powerful, in order to actively confront what has changed in your life, that bothers me. My problem lies with the incumbent narrative that how you choose to live, and ultimately to die, can ever be about losing. Or even that dying might be a choice, or an act of omission. In most contexts the word 'fighter' is, for me, largely a hollow one. I might as well be hearing something as seemingly benign as 'They love to read'.

Actually, I'd prefer to be told that my patient loves to read or has a favourite bench in the park where they like to sit. That at least is the sort of information I can feed constructively into a narrative, and I am a strong advocate of caring about a patient's narrative. If I am ever sick and a doctor finds himself or herself in a situation where they would like to know something else about me, tell them that I like the smell of books, that I like to eat dark chocolate, that sometimes the thought of ever being seriously ill terrifies me, but that at other times

I think I would probably be able to cope. Tell them I spent years of my life as an Irish dancer. Tell them anything at all, apart from 'She's a fighter'.

One day I am standing in a corridor outside a patient's side-room, with three consultants and the patient's friend. The patient is young, in her thirties; she is only partially conscious and is propped up on a pillow. She has gaunt, hollow cheeks and I think, if I asked her to hold her own head up unsupported, her neck would snap under that weight and her head would tumble onto the floor. Her hair is thin and her elbows look far too large to be part of her frame. I am reminded of another patient who had come into the emergency department one evening a few years before. He was in his fifties, emaciated and dying from cancer. When I approached the trolley that he lay on, to speak to him, he spoke slowly in a whisper and asked me if I would mind holding his head up for him while we talked. I stood beside him with one hand scooped underneath his head, raising it up just far enough that he could see me clearly when I spoke to him. That is probably the most humbling thing a patient has ever asked me to do for them, and I cannot bring myself to respect a narrative that reduces the journey of patients like him to the idea of them not being tough enough to survive.

In the case of the young woman now in the side-room, there is actually a chance that intensive care could help her get better so that she could, in the best-case scenario, have a year to live, or more. But the burden of treatment is huge, and we might also simply be sentencing her to a death plugged into our machines.

The consultants have talked back and forth for most of the morning: what is the right thing, the best thing, the kindest thing? What is it that she would want?

We don't know.

There aren't any family members to speak to, but this friend had been nominated as a next of kin, when our patient was more alert. While someone updates the friend on the situation, I watch the patient's wispy frame in the distance. I hear the friend tell us that he understands, adding calmly, 'Look, this isn't a surprise; she isn't really a fighter.'

Before this moment, I do not think I would have believed that anybody would ever say those words to me, and I have consciously to decide if I have heard him correctly.

Then he adds, 'She just hasn't got that in her.'

And I am speechless in the wake of these words; disgusted, honestly, and uncomfortable. I realise there is something worse than hearing that vapid, hollow phrase, which I have come to dislike so much, and it is actually hearing the opposite applied to a dying patient. Inside me, a defensive retaliation boils up. But I know it doesn't matter at all, either way, what I think in that moment. So I stop myself from saying anything.

In the end, we decide to take her to intensive care and she improves, quicker than we had expected. When she is extubated and the medical team comes to discuss plans for what will happen over the next few months, she is thankfully in a place where she can tell us what she would like. She says she wants to go home and live the time that she has left as comfortably as possible, but without escalating treatment or intervention. She asks for palliation and is discharged home. I don't see the friend again.

As a doctor, I have to believe that within the context of my interaction with patients, I will for the most part not give disgust a foothold. I don't claim any state of perfection; a significant amount of this behaviour is motivated by self-preservation. Put simply, behaving any other way would make my job pretty hard to cope with.

When I was a new doctor in A&E, a prisoner was brought into hospital with a fairly simple head-wound requiring stitches. He came with three prison guards in tow, who told my senior that, due to the patient's extremely violent nature and usual behaviour around men, it would be helpful for them if he saw a female doctor, who shouldn't act 'too familiar' with him. I was the chosen one.

My initial thought-process began: 'Why should he get to choose the gender of doctor that he is treated by?' But following soon after this thought, it occurred to me that I often happily oblige a female patient who, for some reason or another, makes a non-malicious request for a female doctor. She might be a patient who is about to seek help for the injuries of domestic abuse, or might tell me she has some problem with intimate discharge. I have not felt any sort of disgust towards their requests for a female presence, so why should I feel any now?

On my way to go and meet this apparently violent man, I was wondering a little about what had happened in his life to create this situation: what crime was he guilty of? But by the time I walked into the room, my overriding thought was that this was a challenge, and I wanted to prove I was capable of establishing a productive relationship with that prisoner-patient. He'd already been judged by the system, which was there for that purpose. It was time now to focus on what my purpose was: to do a neurological assessment, sew up his head and send him on his way.

When it comes to emotions, I am far from robotic, but I have a job to do and there are 'rules', including the ones in the Declaration of Geneva that I stood and attested to at my graduation ceremony:

The health and wellbeing of my patient will be my first consideration [...] I will not permit considerations of age, disease or disability, creed, ethnic origin, gender, nationality, political affiliation, race, sexual orientation, social standing or any other factor to intervene between my duty and my patient.

Consideration of all those things or *'any other factor'* – it's a funny old state of mind, I think, to require of someone that they would not allow *anything* at all *ever* to come between their duty to their patient. Medical professionals do lots of exams, many of which take the format of multiple-choice questions. There is a presumed rule of thumb amongst us that if a possible answer includes something as immovable as 'never' or 'always', it is unlikely to be the correct option. This is because it is unlikely to be compatible with what we know about medicine and disease: that there must always be room for doubt or variation. In medicine, things are almost never 'always' and almost never 'never'.

So while I do proactively try not to give myself the opportunity to feel revulsion towards a patient's background, sometimes it has to be a deliberate process.

Once I looked after a man who had been convicted for rape and murder; his victim had been a woman who was not far off my own age at the time of her demise. I found out his background by accident, from a conversation I overheard on the ward, moments before I was going to meet him. Within the context of the gossip, my colleagues had sounded disgusted, but their whispers were removed in that moment from the patient. They weren't standing in that shared space of a consultation, the space that truly locks your focus into the contract between one patient and one health-care professional.

With this new, unwelcome knowledge, I entered his room and sat on the chair by his bed to do a lumbar puncture. I asked permission, explained the procedure and then I ran my fingers gently along the skin that covered his spine, and felt the warmth of his skin beneath my fingers as I pushed a little harder to mark out the indentation of spaces between his vertebrae. I put one hand on the area just above his upward-facing hip and used the other to wipe his skin with alcohol, before infiltrating it with local anaesthetic. Externally, each step occurred exactly like every other time that I had carried out this procedure. When I had finished with the local anaesthetic, I asked him to let me know if he felt any pain. A challenge: to treat him like everybody else.

Does it mean that I didn't feel any amount of disgust towards him? If I look closely, I suppose I must have felt some repulsion, or I wouldn't now recall the deliberate nature of my intention to treat him the same way as everybody else. Being humane wouldn't be a deliberate or noteworthy action, if I wasn't railing against something.

When you read about crime or domestic abuse, or you see it on the television, you can feel whatever it is you want to feel. All of those who work on the front line of our health service know, though, that in practice, more often than not, treating somebody who you think is probably a criminal or a victim of domestic abuse doesn't leave you with much scope to express any personal emotion at all.

Margaret was in her fifties. She had dry, frizzy hair piled up on top of her head and a face that looked tired in every respect. Her skin was tinged with grey, she had lines around her mouth from smoking and, although it was warm, she wore a huge knee-length, thick beige woollen cardigan over black skinny jeans. She came to A&E because she had a persistent cough and a pain in her chest. She also confided in me that her husband was frequently violent towards her. When I suggested that she needed to stay on the acute medical ward for a few hours, so that we could do a chest X-ray and some other bloods, Margaret panicked and told me that if she wasn't home soon, her husband would come and find her. I told her there were one or two worrisome causes of her symptoms that I needed to exclude, because she had come to me for that reason. Of course I also offered her help for the alleged abuse, and the senior nurse did the same. We gave her the numbers for a refuge and for helplines. We gave her options, but you cannot force an adult to accept help and, you may call it unwise, but wisdom is not a required aspect of mental capacity.

Margaret was admitted to the ward and, as it was the weekend, her workup took longer to arrange than I had expected. When I visited the ward to reassure her that she wouldn't be waiting too much longer, she told me it was too late – her husband had phoned and he was already on his way to pick her up. She told me that when he arrived she would self-discharge. I asked if that was what she wanted to do; she told me that she had to.

He arrived just as I was leaving the bed space. He looked smart, as if he had come from an office job, wearing an open-collared shirt and navy slacks. Before this man made a move to leave with his wife, he found me outside at the nurses' station. I stood up before he reached me. He stopped at the desk, leaned over the counter and told me in a low voice that if he saw me interfering in his business again, he would 'sort me out'.

It's deeply uncomfortable to feel that sort of fear in your job. Outwardly, I told him quite clearly that if he spoke to me like that again, I would call the police. Inwardly, I felt a wreck, and wondered if he knew where I lived or where my car was parked. I felt perhaps one-millionth of the intimidation that Margaret had felt over the course of their relationship, and I couldn't stand it. I couldn't stand that this was her situation. So I told the consultant. I told the charge nurse, and then I phoned our safeguarding team. But their reply was exactly what I already knew: that we can give an adult with mental capacity all the information and advice and options in the world, but we cannot force them to act on it.

Margaret left with that man, and I am sure her situation continued. I think if someone had asked me then what my primary emotion was in the aftermath of that encounter, I'd have said it was closest to despair.

Despair at the reality of sitting down with a woman whose life was everything it should never have been, and not being able to help her. I have become conditioned to centre my feelings that way – it is the most comfortable option.

On the whole, I find it unnatural to judge people without recourse to doubt, and I find it perhaps too easy to take the position of advocate. I am aware this can be an annoying trait, particularly if you just want me to sit and listen while you vent about someone. My will to oppose notions of pure evil can make me a less-than-good listener at times. I find it hard to condemn people, but perhaps the truth is that I have never been in a situation where I have been pushed hard enough.

Once I had three patients who I often wish could have met each other: a British Second World War veteran, a Luftwaffe pilot and a woman who fled Germany in 1940. They all passed through my care within a couple of weeks of each other, which struck me as a strange coincidence. It now strikes me that the opening of this story also sounds like I am about to tell you a bad

'Paddy Englishman, Paddy Scotsman and Paddy Irishman joke'. (I am not.)

The German woman, Agnes, had dementia and cancer, complicated by resulting electrolyte derangement, which worsened her confusion. She was rarely lucid, but one evening when she was, I asked her when she had emigrated to Britain, and she replied in her still-thick accent and through watery and distressed eyes, 'I wasn't a Jew, but I loved one and they were good people. I could not stay and see what they were doing.' I wished she didn't have dementia; I wished I could have sat and learned from all that she could tell me, rather than just catching those intermittent moments of lucidity.

The British war veteran, Harry, was the type of patient who kept all the men talking in his bay. He had a personality that created community, which in the context of long hospital stays for older adults who are waiting on social care or rehabilitation can be invaluable. He told me that he'd been sent home early from the front line in France with a nasty infected dog-bite. He laughed and told me that if he could give me one bit of advice about keeping healthy, it would be not to hang around stray dogs. However, he knew that dog-bite – as his ticket home from the front line – had probably saved his life. That bite gave the world his children and his grandchildren. It also gave me this story.

Derek, the Luftwaffe pilot, was a soldier from Austria who fell out of the sky. Like many in his situation, he was kept as a prisoner-of-war and, like many, he never went 'home' afterwards. When I met Derek, he was dying and he told me he felt grateful for his life; that he felt he'd received more than was owed to him.

I have thought about why this memory is important to me. I am struck by a sense of what a privilege it is to have met these three patients, and by a sense of gratitude for the opportunity I get to see into people's lives, to hear experiences, to hear stories. There are days when I am both humbled by and in awe of the experiences of the patients I am surrounded by.

When I stood by Derek's bed, I was just miles outside a city that had been pummelled by those devastating bomb raids in the Second World War. That devastation had brought people to their knees, and had torn apart families who were still alive and living around me. Yet I could not even imagine a position where I could feel an ounce of revulsion or disgust towards a man who, for all I knew, had formed one of the number carrying out that raid, or one like it. Instead, I felt wonder about how that man had rebuilt his life in an enemy land, and I felt sadness that his lot in life had put him in that plane in the first place. I felt awe. I felt the same level of awe and respect that I had felt speaking with Harry, the British soldier, and Agnes, the German refugee. But what would I have felt, without the hindsight of history and the buffer of time? If I had been a doctor standing by a captured Luftwaffe pilot's bed the day after a blitz in the midst of war? If my house now lay in ruins, if my sister had been blown away?

I am privileged to have existed in a world where my own experience of war has always been indirect and distant – through coverage of current events by news outlets, or through the eyes of a protagonist in a story. In *The Yellow Birds*, ex-soldier Kevin Powers recounts the story of his life after a tour of duty in Afghanistan; he tells us that 'All pain is the same. Only the details are different.' I learned, early on in my journey as a doctor, that this is a useful standpoint from which to see some patients.

When I was still a medical student I spoke with a patient who had presented with symptoms of depression.

Disgust

I was on rotation to a general practice, and this was to be an observed assessment in consultation skills. The GP sat in the corner as I listened to the patient tell me how he felt about his friend's recent death. We spent a long time talking about how he was struggling to cope in the aftermath, about the trouble he had sleeping. Afterwards, when the patient had gone, the GP told me that this man was currently a suspect in the assumed murder of his friend. He told me it had been in all the local papers, and that his friend had been known to the staff at the practice. The GP's idea was that I should carry out the consultation because, as the newcomer without any of that information, I could be the most impartial.

From what was in the public domain, it seemed very possible that this man could have been guilty, and while I was surprised to have learned this had been his context, I wasn't disgusted. Even in retrospect. I was shocked, yes, but I had also heard him tell me how much his life had fallen apart. And when you sit down with one patient and their pain in that situation, there isn't really room for the context of everyone else involved. There isn't a remit for engaging in some sort of world-view ethical construction about whether this person's hurt is now somehow deserved, as retribution for something else. It is of no use to me to engage in such adjudication. As long as there was nobody else who required safeguarding – and there wasn't – it was not my job to act as judge or juror. I was there to train to be a doctor.

I did meet that patient again in consultation, and I am being honest when I say that I really don't think I was disgusted, even then. I didn't follow his trial. The outcome seemed irrelevant to me.

If that victim's mother had come into my surgery and had explained her devastation at the presumed murder of her son, and she'd told me that his friend was being considered a prime suspect, I am sure I would have found it quite easy to feel disgust towards the man accused. Towards the man who wasn't my patient.

I take myself through these kinds of thought-experiments because I would like to know that I am capable of feeling some disgust in these situations. Despite the rules of professionalism, it seems to me an important part of being human, to feel and react to these things.

I have wondered if this job sometimes takes part of that away from me. The cult of medicine can feel overwhelming at times. 'I solemnly pledge to consecrate my life to the service of humanity' – did you know that the Declaration of Geneva says that, too? I have apparently promised not just to devote my working life or my professional career to the service of humanity, but to consecrate my life, without further qualification, to that service. On the morning of graduation, when I stood in a cap and gown and recited those words together with a room full of my classmates, I was, I think, caught up in the romanticism of it all. In retrospect, those words seem pretty intense, and it is clear why colleagues sometimes say that being a doctor often feels like being part of a religion or a cult. This job makes demands on all aspects of your life and character. The standards to which we are bound weave their way into every part of your life, so that eventually you don't really know where those standards end and your own ones begin. The adult I became in my twenties lived a life that was dominated by notions of who I was told a doctor was supposed to be. Would I be a different adult, if had chosen a different career?

It has not yet been two years since graduation and I am standing on a ward, looking at a parent who has been accused of harming their five-year-old child. The child will die, I am already sure of this. The parent volunteers, in a flustered tone, that they haven't 'done anything wrong', and I reply that it is not my job to judge; I am here to do my best for the child, and the police and child-protection services are obliged to investigate. The extended family arrive and they are angry – not really at me, but they need to be angry at somebody, so their frustration navigates in my direction. They tell me we are adding to their pain.

I look at that beautiful boy, lying inanimate on a child-sized bed with his limbs spread, tethered to our pumps with various lines, and I realise what I have said to them might not be a lie. I had this strange feeling in that moment that it might actually be true: I really wasn't passing judgement. And I suddenly feel disgusted with myself.

I am sitting feet away from this little boy, and I honestly think the parent could be responsible for their impending death. I want to feel outraged. I want to bubble over with horror. I want to feel the disgust that I might feel if I had read this story in the newspaper. I want to throw lightning and explode dynamite. I want to make noise on behalf of the innocence that was lost, but I cannot. It is there somewhere, the outburst, but it is only a hoarse whisper hidden somewhere in a corner inside me, and within the walls of this hospital all that I can process and output is a bottom line: that I should do my job.

That professionalism felt uncomfortable to me – for the first time it felt I was perhaps being asked not to be human. Humane: yes, maybe, but less of a human for it?

Then I wave those thoughts out of my head and hope that I am still human, after all.

Hope

There is a crack in everything.
That's how the light gets in.

Leonard Cohen, 'Anthem'

CLAIRE WAS FORTY-EIGHT YEARS old. She was 5 feet nothing and weighed less than 45kg, with a host of chronic
conditions to her name. One of those was end-stage renal
failure. Unfortunately, some of her other problems meant
that Claire would not now be able to have a kidney transplant and would always require regular haemodialysis.*

* The kidneys are, amongst other things, responsible for getting
rid of certain toxins and controlling the balance of fluid and elec-
trolytes, such as potassium, in our bodies. When somebody has
end-stage renal failure, haemodialysis involves passing blood from
the person through a machine that takes care of these jobs, before
pumping it back into them. For most, this happens three times a
week for about three hours at a time, and it is very possible to live a
full and active life while also being reliant on haemodialysis.

When I was still a very junior doctor on a renal ward, Claire had a complex episode of ill health and stayed with us as an inpatient for more than three months. There was a photo by her bed that showed her sitting in a garden with her friends in the summer; they were laughing, drinking Prosecco around a white plastic table, and I suspect were heading for a night out. I didn't recognise that Claire in the photograph. But when I looked at how her brown roots now contrasted with the dyed blonde of her shoulder-length hair, it reminded me that she really used to be somebody different. Somebody who got her hair done, who woke up in the morning, looked in her wardrobe and chose what she wanted to wear. Somebody who sat in her kitchen and had breakfast, but who occasionally just grabbed a coffee on the run. Somebody who *could* run. Now her body looked like it ought to belong to somebody who had seen many more decades on this planet than she had. The long hospital stay had robbed her of much of her remaining muscle mass and she had become frail; her thighs had shrunk, her calves had all but disappeared. She struggled to get out of bed. I had yet to see Claire stand up by herself or mobilise to the bathroom, or into a chair unaided.

Aside from basic ward-reviews, a lot of my day-to-day chat with Claire at that time was about encouraging her to participate in rehabilitation and physiotherapy and, in some ways, about helping her to look forward into the future. One day the nurse had mentioned to me that Claire seemed down, and more disengaged than usual. I had coincidentally that morning signed a request form for some specific shoes, which the occupational therapy and orthotics department felt would help her with rehabilitation. I went to see Claire on my round and, without giving it a great deal of thought, said to her enthusiastically, 'I've heard you're about to step up and get moving more! And you'd better, because I signed an order for a pair of shoes for you today.'

'Really?' she asked, perking up in the bed just enough to make it noticeable.

'Yes, so now you know: you've got shoes to fill!'

More than a week passed without giving much more thought to that exchange, until one afternoon I walked back onto the ward and the sister in charge, spotting me, said with a smile, 'Go and see Claire, she's been waiting to tell you something.' When Claire saw me come towards her, she was alive and animated as I had never seen her before. She looked almost as if she really could be the person in that photograph next to her. Sitting up in her pink hospital nightdress, with her thin arms outstretched to me from her bed, she said in a shaking voice, 'I stood up.'

I hugged Claire and she felt like a delicate bird in my arms. I saw myself like an overbearing toddler who had picked up a kitten to give it a cuddle, making the adults in the room wince and say, 'Don't squeeze it too tightly!' I told her how proud I was of her achievement; how proud she should be of herself. If that moment hadn't happened, I don't think I would have ever guessed how happy that news of Claire standing up could have made me.

I wish I could tell you now that Claire went from strength to strength and went home, but the truth is that she died in hospital a few months later and she never put on those shoes. When I think about her now, it is hard not to wonder what it meant to her when I announced that she had shoes to fill: Did I ask her to hope for a future that wasn't there? Was I in any way partly responsible for raising her hopes? And if I was, was it okay that she never put those shoes on in the end?

Hope

When I tell a patient, 'Hey, I think you can do it', does the inevitable imbalance of power in that situation mean they are more likely to think something is possible? Perhaps that's self-flattery and you might think: Well, *there* is a doctor with an inflated sense of self-importance. But I believe that every ounce of strength it took for Claire to stand came from her. She was responsible for the combined force of muscle and mind that it required to place her feet, firmly, on the cold, unforgiving hospital floor and push her weight down through them. But I wonder what my role was, in igniting the hope behind her strength.

Doctors are expected to deal in evidence-based medicine. We deal in statistics, in defined confidence intervals around an estimate of something. I had absolutely no firm evidence base that Claire would actually stand on her feet again. I had no real evidence that she would use those shoes. I believed there was some unquantifiable possibility, but I honestly never stopped to think how small that possibility might have been. What's more, it wasn't even enough to make me at all surprised that in the end she died. I had really hoped Claire would get back on her feet, and I wanted her to feel that hope, too. I don't know if that is okay.

Hope is tricky. Within the context of medicine, it is the trickiest thing that I know of. And before we get any further, I should admit here and now that I don't understand it. It seems cruel that I have known my own hope to swell to its maximal size in the midst of loss, longing or impending grief. It is when I feel most emptiness, or I have most reason to doubt, that hope arrives and tries to fill the black hole. Hope in the absence of surety. I let it in and I know that if the hole were not so deep or so black, I would not need to summon so much hope to fill it. I have come to realise that the more hope that I require to fill a void, conversely the less hopeful I should probably be. If we were logical, that is what we would know: hope is only really important when we have good reason to be hopeless. Anything else would surely be solved with something different: certainty, anticipation, ambition, confidence, conviction or self-belief?

Recently, there was a young man called Andy. He had been brought into intensive care following an out-of-hospital cardiac arrest, and I cannot tell you why this happened to him, because we never really found out. He was younger than me and had recently returned from a year working and travelling in Thailand. He had proposed to his girlfriend on a beach before they returned, and she now sat, with his parents, anxiously by his bedside. I could still see the tan-line on his wrist from where he had worn a leather-cuffed bracelet. It was the sort of item you only really buy on holidays, and I could picture him wearing it on the beach and in the bars. We had taken it off after he arrived. I had put an arterial line in that wrist.

For this particular sort of non-shockable, out-of-hospital cardiac arrest, the crude survival to some form of hospital discharge has been quoted as being as low as 2 per cent. That's two patients in every 100.

Just two? Yes.

Do I mean that 98 per cent could be expected to die? Yes, and 2 per cent could be expected to live.

But I could also tell you that two people in 100 is the equivalent of twenty in every 1,000; 200 in every 10,000; or 2,000 in 100,000. If I make the denominator big enough, you can arrive at a picture of 2,000 people, alive and standing in front of you. It suddenly feels more possible that your loved one's familiar face will peer back at you from that actually rather large crowd of 2,000 faces, and you will forget that there are 98,000 people on the other side of those odds. You will embrace hope and forget the denominator.

From the outset, the odds were stacked against Andy; his odds of not surviving were definitely more than 90 per cent, but because I see so many cardiac arrests, I can also sometimes temporarily forget the denominator. Often it is important that I do so; doctors need to remain attentive enough not to miss the clues that might tell us this patient could be in the minority.

Throughout the first day I spent looking after him, I found more than one potentially positive sign: Andy was triggering his own breaths on the ventilator; he had required less and less blood pressure support; he had required a minimal amount of extra oxygen through the ventilator; and his renal function tests had remained normal. I wrote some of these things down in my morning review, without consciously ascribing to them any real hope or meaning. I don't think I actually knew how hopeful I had let myself become until around half-past seven in the evening, when I picked up the phone to return a page. The ICU nurse on the other end of the line told me, 'It's Andy, his pupils have just blown.' 'Blown', in this sense, is a word that means intractably dilated.

I hurried back to the unit, calling the consultant on my way. We stabilised Andy as best we could, before transporting him together to the CT scanner to obtain some up-to-date images of his head. It was unspoken between us that what we were about to see was a swollen and damaged brain; a brain that had been deprived of oxygen for too long at the point of arrest and would soon cease to function. Undoubtedly we both expected it. We wheeled Andy into the scan room, transferred him across onto the table, checked that all his lines, cables and monitors were in a safe position, and then sat on the other side of the glass screen to observe while Andy moved in and out of the CT scanner. The expected occurred, and yet the consultant, who had been in this situation many more times than me, seemed no less deflated by this exceedingly probable turn of events. As the scan came to an end, and without turning away from the glass screen between the patient and us, he said flatly, out loud, but almost to himself, 'I really allowed myself to hope on this one.'

The next day I saw the pre-hospital emergency-medicine doctor who had retrieved Andy from the community, and I told her the sad news that he had died. 'You know, I think we all really had a good feeling about that one,' I said, when she expressed her disappointment.

'But they were always slim chances, weren't they?' she replied. 'We knew that, we just got over-excited when we thought he might be the exception.'

She was right. We had hoped because, subconsciously, we clung to things that suggested Andy could be the exception, not because the odds ever really suggested that he would be. We'd looked for the positives – from one perspective, it looked promising, but from most others, it was clear there was little reason to hope.

Some of my more senior colleagues have told me that, for a doctor, hope is not just tricky; it is dangerous, because it equates to emotional investment, which often leads to grief. They say that you cannot constantly expose yourself to that much emotional risk, as there would simply be too many patients, too many adverse outcomes to contend with. The consultants who tell me this are not the sort of nihilistic people whom you might associate with such a statement. They are, for the most part, the ones that I would see as caring; the ones that I would like to emulate. These consultants aren't the sorts of doctors that I would associate with taking their heart out of their practice. But I think the reason they caution me is because, really, they do the same, too.

When I encounter a consultant whose sadness seems to be not just about the youth and vitality lost to death, but about hope spent and lost, it tells me that even the most seasoned doctor will allow hope to sneak up uninvited and take a seat. It tells me that there will always be cracks in the façade of our logic; and yes, we will let the light slip through these cracks; we will let the light fill a space greater than anything that was ever owed to it.

It also tells me that, when it comes to hope, doctors are not very different from those to whom we break our news, from those to whom we try and explain the odds. So I don't think I can truly regret that I had invested in hope for Andy, or for the many patients like him who have passed through my hands and similarly met their demise, entirely in accordance with the odds. If Andy had been in the minority and had survived, I might have looked back now and felt that I knew he would make it all along.

I think that despite our attempts at seeming otherwise, doctors do remain vulnerable to hope. But the difference is that usually we don't visibly share it. When you stand beside your relative, with your hand resting on theirs and tell yourself, 'I hope they pull through – I know they'll pull through', I hope that, too. Often, I am simply hoping that in another room.

Pat was a husband and a father of grown-up children. He was a bricklayer who'd had an accident at work, falling from some scaffolding on a building site and ending up with a complex, traumatic brain injury. We admitted him to the intensive-care unit and for more than forty days he did not get any better; in fact he got worse. Slowly Pat became this entity whose physiology we couldn't control. He became somebody that we struggled to ventilate, could not wean off sedation and could not 'wake up'.

Over the course of those weeks, Pat's personhood appeared to sink down further and further inside him, until eventually it felt as if nobody on the team could picture him transitioning from our care and finally achieving the goal of being discharged home. We were patient, but day after day passed, the bed beside his turned over five or six different patients during his stay, and ultimately the time came when we had to sit down and address the elephant in the room: where was this going?

We gathered Pat's family and told them there was a very significant chance that we would not be able to wean him from the support of intensive care. We told them we regretted it immensely, but as more time passed, things seemed less and less salvageable. We told them the most likely outcome now would not be favourable. The conversation was done carefully and with compassion; its purpose was always to share our thoughts with Pat's family, to keep them part of the conversation. None of the doctors I know walk into conversations with relatives to try and convince them they have a crystal ball, but it was important that the family tempered their hope.

The following morning I walked past Pat's bay, where his wife, Linda, stood leaning on the bed rail and holding her husband's hand. She saw me and gestured hurriedly for me to come over. 'I know,' she began, 'I know what was discussed yesterday, but he's different today. Don't you think he's different?'

At that moment, Pat's daughter also arrived. 'Hello, Mum,' she said, taking off her cardigan. Then, spotting me, she paused and added warily, 'Oh, has something happened?'

Much of the time, in this kind of situation, the patient is not markedly changed at all and the differences that people feel they can see cannot be ascribed any definitive prognostic value. But this time it was different. Pat, although not sedated, lay there as I had always known him to; he didn't move, and the ventilator pushed air in and out of his tracheostomy – but his eyes were open.

Not just open, they were tracking his wife and his daughter. Flicking between them, as if screaming, 'I am here.' He was there.

'Don't you think he's different?' Linda prompted me again, nervously.

I tried to think quickly. What did it mean that Pat had opened his eyes? It did not mean for certain that he would get off the ventilator, or regain a semblance of who he was. It might not change a thing.

Seconds passed, as Linda and her daughter stared expectantly at me in my silence, both of their faces begging me for hope.

In those seconds I was asking myself how much hope I could reasonably give them. Misplaced hope often

seems the most unkind thing you can give a family. It is
hard enough to suggest that the time is coming to make
some difficult decisions. But once you deliver that blow –
once you give a family all the information you actually
have, and watch them leave the room deflated, knowing
they will lie on their pillows, eyes wide, trying to come
to terms with what you have said – it makes it harder
to risk telling them that the unexpected has happened.
It isn't because I don't want to be wrong; it is because
I can think of few responsibilities greater than handing somebody hope. Linda wasn't asking my opinion
because she wanted to know if I agreed that Pat's eyes
appeared to be following us. She was asking me because
I was a doctor, and she wanted to know what it meant.

I considered my options and settled on an answer: 'I
have never seen his eyes open like that, no.'

It was a feeble and ineffectual agreement, a statement from someone sitting well and truly on the fence. I
told them that I would arrange a new meeting for them
with neurosurgery and intensive care.

When I walk back into the office and relay the details
of what I have just seen to the other registrar, I am buoy-
ant with that news. I am hopeful, I can feel it welling up

inside me. The vision of those quietly screaming eyes. The idea that Pat might be 'the one' – the minority. I can feel the rush of pleasure from knowing that this is why intensive care exists, and maybe we can help. I hope, I hope, I hope.

But to expose my own human tendency to hope at this stage would be to see it magnified tenfold in Linda's eyes. I fear even a small amount of that light will ignite a fire. I fear, because I have no idea yet what the future holds, and although Linda is not my patient, in intensive care we must often hold relatives as an extension of those whom we are treating. I know my new-found optimism risks doing her harm, and I know the rule: *Primum non nocere* (First, do no harm). So when I stand with Linda, I push my hope down inside me. I wait for more evidence and think perhaps I might share it tomorrow, or the next day. I will share my hope when I have something more tangible than hope to offer her.

Two weeks later, Pat was sitting on the edge of the bed. He could manage without a ventilator and he liked to listen to Sinatra. His face was as it had always been, but it had become entirely different to me, because I could see his face so differently now. Perhaps that is what surprised me the most: that I had unknowingly let his face slip away, swamped beneath the darkness of his journey this far.

Two weeks later still, Pat was sitting in a large, high armchair. This chair is used for patients who are just beginning to sit out in intensive care and it is a cumbersome construction. Sitting in this enormous chair, Pat dominated the centre of his bay. He slowly looked around, seemingly surveying his new kingdom – this strange place that he had unexpectedly come to reside in – and I remember telling him that he looked like a king on a throne. Over the course of those weeks, every single one of Pat's seemingly small achievements made me so happy: our King of Hope.

It is no secret that doctors aren't always right when we give a prognosis, but when we're wrong I believe we are as happy as anybody else. Most intensive-care doctors I meet tell me that they would rather give realistic odds, even if they are pessimistic, and risk that patient being the minority who 'make it', than be responsible for somebody's false hope. I find myself annoyed when I hear stories presented in the media as doctors pessimistically trying to dash hopes – the headlines read,

'Patient defies doctors who gave her a 10 per cent chance of survival' or 'Doctors gave me three months, and twenty years later I'm still proving them wrong'. It is not that we did not want you to hope; we just had an obligation to give you what we saw as the facts. And unless we actually said we were 100 per cent sure that something would happen, there was always a chance. The odds may have been dreadful, but we were still on your side. If I tell you there is a 1 per cent chance that your mother will make it out of hospital and then she makes it, I will always be pleased that she was among the 1 per cent. The 1 per cent makes me get out of bed in the morning. The 1 per cent is why I can do this job.

The thing about odds is that they only tell you about a large sample group. If you are the patient, the odds don't really matter; what matters is whether *your* outcome is favourable. I remember sitting in an office with a woman, her husband and a consultant neurosurgeon. I was still in my second year of practice, and I was taking notes while the consultant was talking her through the consent form for a biopsy of her brain tumour, which would happen later that day. 'Informed consent' requires that a patient is abreast of the risks: not just the adverse effects that we think are likely, but the rare ones, too. The ones that probably won't happen, but still might. The consultant told the woman that he could also try and debulk some of the tumour's mass, which might be helpful in the long run, but because of her tumour's location, this would potentially also risk damaging her ability to speak. The odds the patient was given were an estimate, and I cannot remember the exact figure now, but for the sake of this story, let's say that opting for some debulking of her tumour increased her risk of speech impairment fivefold, to about 20 per cent. What the consultant said to her next has always stayed with me: 'The odds of this happening are small, but I really need you to understand that if it happens to you, 20 per cent is irrelevant; you and your life will be affected. The odds won't matter any more.'

I became acutely aware of what we were asking this patient to do: to make a decision about how exactly she would like to gamble. To have her tumour debulked, or just have a small biopsy and hope that the histopathology results suggested it was not aggressive, or that other treatments would be available. The consultant said he could not make this decision for her; it was up to her to decide her comfortable level of risk. The patient opted to ask the consultant to debulk whatever amount of the tumour he could, and as I watched the ink flow out of the pen onto the dotted line at the end of the consent form, I felt that, more than anything else, her signature must be a record of hope.

Of course we record it as 'informed consent', but how informed can a gamble ever really be? We give patients access to odds and statistics in good faith, but when it comes down to signing on the dotted line, what we are often asking our patients to do is just hope. Hope that they can trust the team; hope that they don't experience the rare complications; hope the odds fall in their favour.

When dealing with patients at the extremes of life, there is an onus on doctors to be alert for the time when the burden of treatment outweighs the expected benefit for a patient. It is imperative that medicine knows when it is time to work *with* death, if it is to work at all. Intensive care, perhaps more than any other speciality, is defined by this specific sort of responsibility. Friends ask me why I have chosen to work in intensive care;

they say, 'What can be worse than seeing so many of your patients die in the end?' But, for me, the difficult reality to bear is not that people die, but that they might die without dignity. If I turn my back on all of the death and shattered hope to which this job exposes me, it will still exist. If I stick around, maybe I can help. So when I become a consultant, I already know that my career will not ultimately be defined by heroic procedures or clever diagnoses. My seniority will be defined by my ability to think ethically, to communicate well and to put my patient at the centre of every decision I make.

Am I keeping this patient alive because I think they will get back to a quality of life that would have been acceptable to them? ... or just because I can keep them 'alive'? ... or because somebody else wants me to? ... or, worse, because I'm too reluctant to have a difficult conversation?

In intensive care, we often engage ourselves in the grossly incongruous charge of informing hope: *Please do hope, but also here – have this helpful information on exactly what the chances are.*

There was a woman with pancreatitis. She had been with us for a few days when one of the nurses came to me, worried that her family did not have a realistic idea of what her chances of survival were. Pancreatitis is one of those conditions that seems a bit bizarre. As an organ, the pancreas has never garnered much celebrity status, and I suppose if I wasn't a doctor I would think, 'So my pancreas is inflamed – how big a deal can it be?' Pancreatitis can be a massive deal; a massive, fatal deal. Since admission, this patient had progressively deteriorated, developing multiple other organ failures. I arranged a family update for later that day.

When the time came, the nurse and I sat down with them. I rehashed to her grown-up children the diagnosis of severe pancreatitis; I took them through their mother's failure to improve; and, as was my intention, I made it very clear that the chances of her dying in the next few days were much higher than the chances of her surviving.

Her daughter, Alex, started to sob and asked with a mixture of frustration and anger, 'So should I hope at all? What is the point in all of *this*?'

This I understood to mean the ventilator, the renal filtration machine, the recurrent courses of antibiotics for superimposed infections, the drugs to keep the patient's blood pressure stable, the one we added when that failed, and the one after that. The central venous lines that we had put in her neck and then her groin, the catheter, the intravenous nutrition. The waiting – also the waiting.

It wasn't that I wanted Alex or her brothers to cry, but I had embarked on that conversation to give them a realistic view of their mother's position. They clearly now seemed to grasp that the situation was dire, and so I could say I had achieved what I had set out to. Mission accomplished?

For me, the often inconvenient reality is that unless I have entered a room to tell a person that their relative is definitively, absolutely dying or dead, it would never be within my remit to bid them not to hope. So, my hands are tied. I answered Alex that of course I wasn't telling her not to hope at all. I replied that if I didn't think there was any chance at all, then we wouldn't continue with this invasive treatment. I said yes, there was a chance she might survive, but it was exceedingly small, and we felt it was important that they understood how sick their mum really was.

Emily Dickinson made a bird called Hope famous. In '"Hope" is the thing with feathers', she tells us about the creature that remains perched inside us, steadfast through all our trials. There is a line that sometimes enters my head: the bird 'sings the tune without the words'. I often wonder if perhaps she meant that hope wasn't interested in the words; not interested in the details, the statistics or the evidence. That maybe the bird just needs a crumb of something, and it will sing as if you have given it an entire loaf to feast upon. Within the context of some of my work, there are times when I am not sure how helpful this little bird actually is.

When we went back to their mum's bedside, Alex gulped back her sob and wiped her face, roughly, with the sleeve of her jumper. Somewhere inside her the bird called Hope feasted on the crumb I had dropped. She brightened and said, with an air of determination, 'She can do it.' Then she sat back down, exactly where she had been before our conversation had happened.

My seniors have told me that in the days or weeks that lie between critical illness and death, relatives will ultimately default to whatever amount of hope they were always going to default to, irrespective of what you tell them.

I walked away and positioned myself at the nurses' station, so I could document our conversation in the notes. I made it clear that I had told them the prognosis was very poor. Looking at those relatives from across the room, I have no idea what value there really was in the documentation of that fact. But in medicine, we are reminded repeatedly, 'If you didn't document it, it didn't happen.' The overwhelming majority of medical complaints that are successful in receiving a monetary payout involve a failure of medical record-keeping. So I made my record of 'I told you so', and I wondered whether I should have stopped talking when the sobbing started. Alex's mum died two days later.

We often sit like this at the boundary between what is life and death. As doctors, it is paramount that we aim to keep the individual patient at the centre of everything we do, but that can be difficult to achieve with certainty in intensive care – it is not at all unusual for me to be present for a patient's entire hospital journey, but to have absolutely no hope of knowing what they are thinking. As your doctor, I can pull the curtains around your bed, say, 'Hello my name is ...' and then, approaching you, pull back the sheet from the upper part of your body as I announce, without expecting a response, 'I am just going to examine your chest.' I can touch your flesh and pull back your eyelids and press my finger onto your sternum for three seconds, to watch your skin slowly fill with colour again. I can listen to the noises that come from inside your lungs, your heart, your abdomen. I can look at your observations and at the monitors that surround you and attempt to guess if, at least, you are not in any pain. I can have an off-by-heart knowledge of exactly what the values of all of the various biochemical markers that we study in your blood are on any particular day. I could talk out loud to you for days and days, but if you are both intubated and sedated on a ventilator, I still will not know what is going on in your mind – if there is anything at all. And you might never even know my name.

My parents always taught me that it is what lies on the inside that counts; but for many of my patients, 'what counts' is – for reasons of sedation, illness or injury – simply locked away. Modern medicine has created these often morally complex situations. Sometimes I look at my patients and wonder how I can ever hope to actually understand or define who they are, without the ability to see so much of what really counts about them. These patients are anything, nothing, everything.

Of course, as doctors we do our best to find ways around trying to understand who a patient is. I can speak to family members and garner some sort of background knowledge and perception of what a patient holds important to them. I can hope they have formed some sort of advance directive, regarding their wishes in situations of extremis, but none of that can ever fully emulate a person or their autonomy. None of that tells us what that person is now – who they are. Mostly, we aim to do what is the least restrictive option, until we can achieve some sort of relationship with the patient in question. If that is a possibility at all.

Within the world of quantum mechanics there is a theory called the 'Copenhagen interpretation'. In very basic terms, this hypothesis states that an object in any sort of physical system can exist in all of its possible forms until observation forces it into a single state (a bit like a boggart in the Harry Potter books).

The Nobel Prize-winning physicist Erwin Schrödinger claimed that the Copenhagen interpretation was flawed. To illustrate why, he came up with a thought-experiment: a cat is placed inside a sealed box with a device that has a precisely 50 per cent chance of killing the cat within an hour. At the end of the hour, what is the state of the cat? Without opening the box, you could not know that the cat was alive, but neither could you say that it was dead. So was it both?

Schrödinger's cat became famous: the cat that was both dead and alive. Sometimes I think that intensive care is home to many such cats.

I am reminded of this when I look at my patient. She's about my age. I place my hand on her wrist and it is warm, but there is no pulse. The arterial line confirms this, because she does not have the classic waveform that would tell me blood is being pumped in a pulsatile manner from her heart, through her arteries. What I see is an ever so vaguely undulating red line, making its way across the monitor. I place my stethoscope on her chest and I cannot hear clear heart sounds. Her chest moves up and down with the ventilator and there are large cannulas, which look more like pipes, running out of her body, taking blood down into a machine, feeding it through an oxygenator and pumping it continuously back into her body.

Her own heart doesn't currently function in any true sense of the word. It had stopped in earnest some days ago, so you could say that she had died, but a team pushed up and down on her chest until the machine was ready to use. And you could say that resuscitation failed, because her heart remained in a non-perfusing rhythm[*] but then she was in the right place, so to speak, and the team had timely access to this machine and some cardiac pacing wires. So, she had a chance. Now she's lying here, her blood being pushed around her body by the pump in the machine next to me. She is deeply sedated. Deeply disconnected from anything that I can definitively identify as life. She is galaxies – light years – away.

I turn to the consultant and ask, 'So we just wait?'

'Yes, we wait to see if her heart will beat functionally again.'

Schrödinger's point was that his cat couldn't possibly be *both* dead and alive. He was illustrating that the Copenhagen interpretation couldn't hold for large organisms, because how could a cat ever simultaneously be both dead and alive?

---

[*]A non-perfusing rhythm is used to describe a situation where the heart has some sort of electrical activity, but the movement of the heart muscle that results from the electrical activity does not allow the heart to do its job as a pump. Blood is still not perfused around the body.

Yet I stare now at Schrödinger's patient: dead or alive?

And I cannot answer that question. I just cannot make up my mind what the answer to this basic question is. And it is not only because this situation is so new to me that I cannot even comprehend this patient's state of being. I know that if I stood at the bedside of a hundred patients like her, I would never truly be able to understand their status: who are they in that moment, and what form do they take? So I default to what I see my patient's relatives default to: time will tell, there is nothing left to do but hope that the coin falls the right way up. Roll the dice, but try not to roll a six. Hope, because I don't know what else to fill that space with, and it is as yet too early to consider making any other decisions.

Four days later, when I look up at the cardiac monitor, it is now tracing an intrinsic heart rate of 100 beats per minute. Familiar, regular; sinus rhythm, a heartbeat that is her own. I place my stethoscope onto her chest, for no other reason than feeling obliged to do her the service of acknowledging that there is something there inside her. To show her that I had made up my mind, that I knew the answer to the question.

It is a ritual; to show her that respect, I listen.

I hear the clear and familiar sound of heart valves opening and closing: lub-dub, lub-dub, lub-dub. I am, I am, I am.

Alive.

I had stood beside her and asked myself: What are the chances? I told myself, 'Slim, very slim.'

We decide to support this wisp of a chance, because the best assessment we can conduct tells us that it is in the patient's best interests. So she is passed from the emergency department team to theatres. She makes her way that day through the hands of surgeons and anaesthetists, nurses, healthcare assistants, radiographers, porters – all of these hands at different times; many more hands to come; and now mine. I do my job and, in the interim, having nothing else to counteract the blind uncertainty, I hope. I hope that she will make it, and I hope that she will be okay with what we did to get her to that point.

Her family ask how things are looking. My face is serious and I tell them what I can be sure of: that we have had a positive sign, but that the bigger picture remains very similar. That she is very sick and that, as we discussed before, there is a significant chance of further complications, underlying brain damage or that what we are doing will not work. But we are doing the best we can.

They hope. I hope. Doing the best we can.

Three weeks later, this patient is not just biologically alive, but is resoundingly, tangibly alive. She has intact brain function and no further need for other organ support. On the day when she is to be discharged to the ward, I pop into her room and wish her luck. As these words come out of my mouth, I can feel something that doesn't happen all that often. I can feel a warm heat rising inside my throat and up into my cheeks. I can feel the hint of tears gathering around my eyes, and I know exactly what this is – because I am the sort of person who cries at happy endings.

I don't cry, nor do I want to, so I keep it short. I say, 'Goodbye, best of luck' and I smile. I want that smile to say something, for it to say: 'You are significant to me.'

She says, 'Thank everyone for looking after me.'

I shake my head to indicate that there is no need for thanks, and reply, 'Of course, that is what we are all here for.'

And as I shut the door and walk away, I consider that she has decades of life ahead of her. I have no idea what her future holds. But I hope that she gets to enjoy it.

Afterword

> Remember, remember, this is now, and now, and now.
> Live it, feel it, cling to it.
>
> Sylvia Plath, *The Journals of Sylvia Plath 1950–1962*

ADULTS HAVE ALWAYS BEEN preoccupied with asking children what they want to be when they grow up. When I was three, Santa Claus brought me a nurse's uniform. The following Christmas, I asked Santa Claus to bring me a pram and a He-Man figurine to put in it. If you're not familiar with this particular 1980s comic-book hero, he was an almost completely naked man who was billed as having superhuman strength, super-speed and indestructible skin. I presume I looked strange next to the other girls on my street, who proudly transported and cared for their plastic babies and dolls, each of them crafted with placid faces, pink lips and rosy cheeks. I don't really know what possessed a four-year-old me to want to take that hero of apparent masculinity, cover him with a blanket and push him around in my pram or include him in my games. But I know what I would have told you I wanted to 'be' when I grew up, if you'd asked me.

From the point when I was really old enough to have some understanding of what a job is, I would have told you I wanted to be a doctor. I suppose you could say that has always been my 'dream job', but now that I have at least partially grown up, I am not really sure what a dream job is supposed to look like, after all. It is probably the case that it doesn't actually *look* like anything, it just *feels* like something; and I wonder what I might have answered, had somebody ventured to ask me at any point, what I expected 'being a doctor' to feel like.

Perhaps you might think I will finish this account by telling you that if I love my job, it is the truly positive experiences and outcomes that, in the end, make it all worthwhile. But that's not it.

I think the majority of adults who have the luxury of not honestly having to fear for their basic safety, immediate health or source of food and shelter will tell you that their wish in life is to be 'happy'. I love my job and yes, it is a job that makes me happy. But it is also a job that can make me immensely sad – and that can make me feel every single emotion around and in between.

I think, as people, part of the beauty of our uniqueness comes from that fact that we are the product of all our experiences, not simply the ones that we have been conditioned to think of as more palatable. So, when I look around at my patients and their families, or flick back inside my own head through the patients and stories that have become not just a part of my memories, but really a part of my own process of 'growing up', it is my intention that I should appreciate them all.

Anybody who works in the health service will tell you that within the walls of a hospital you cannot hide from the realities of life. Life is everywhere: it is around every corner, in every bed and on every chair in the waiting room. Life comes to me etched in wrinkles and scars, dampened by tears and lightened by jokes. Life comes to me interwoven with infection, trauma, cancer, suicide, frailty, chronic disease, rehabilitation, death and everything in between, and it does not have a filter.

What I experience each day alongside colleagues, patients and their families could never be justifiably defined as merely joy in spite of fear, or hope in spite of anger, or any other emotion. It is simply joy *and* hope, anger *and* fear, disgust, distraction and grief – we all slide from one of these feelings to another in a moment, and this is what we share and what makes us engaged with the world around us.

So that is where I have to stand at the beginning of every shift: ready to experience each of these emotions as they come, and hoping that because, like my patients, I cannot hope to hide from them, perhaps I might appreciate each emotion as an opportunity to know what it really means to be alive.

So if you ask a partially grown-up me now what being a doctor really feels like, I will tell you that I think the answer is simple: being a doctor feels like *feeling* everything.

Acknowledgements

I WOULD LIKE TO say thank you:

To the then neurosurgical registrar who, almost seven years ago, gifted his senior house-officer a book by Frank Vertosick and, in doing so, introduced me to the concept that I might also have stories to tell. To Neil Hallows, editor for the British Medical Association, who not long afterwards received, unsolicited, my first 'story' and has been an incredible source of guidance and support to me ever since.

To all the colleagues I have worked with. To the consultants and mentors whose doors I have always been able to knock on. To my peers, nurses and members of the wider healthcare team who have supported me along the way.

To my big brother, whose presence in my life gave me an opportunity to learn some of the things that medical school could never teach me. To my wonderful sisters. To my parents, to whom I owe more than I could ever acknowledge, and who allowed me to believe not only that I could do anything I wanted to work hard enough to achieve, but also that whatever I wanted to do was okay.

To the friends who have loved and supported me throughout all this.

To Anna-Sophia Watts, an editor at Penguin Random House, who one day invited me for lunch and has put up with me, admirably, ever since.

To the books I have read.

To Spa Town Coffee, a place where I sat and wrote so much of this book.

And to the patients – most sincerely to the patients.

Thank you, all.

Quotation Acknowledgements

p.vii: 'IX. The Four Ages of Man', *Supernatural Songs*, in *'Parnell's Funeral' and other poems* (1935) by W. B. Yeats, from *Collected Poems*, Vintage, 1992.

p.9: *Long Walk to Freedom* by Nelson Mandela, Abacus, 1994. Copyright © Nelson Rolihlahla Mandela 1994. Reprinted with the permission of Little, Brown Book Group.

p.20: *The Lifted Veil* by George Eliot, Oxford University Press, 1921.

p.49: *Grief is the Thing with Feathers* by Max Porter, Faber & Faber, 2015. Copyright © Max Porter 2015.

p.75: 'Late Fragment', from *All Of Us* by Raymond Carver published by Harvill Press. Reproduced by permission of The Random House Group Ltd. © 1996.

p.89: *The Ocean at the End of the Lane* by Neil Gaiman, Headline, 2013. Copyright © Neil Gaiman 2013.

p.97: 'Of Tolling Bell I Ask the Cause', by Emily Dickinson, from *The Poems of Emily Dickinson*, edited by Ralph W. Franklin, Harvard University Press, 2005.

p.109: 'Fight Song', co-written by Rachel Platten and Dave Bassett, Columbia Records.

p.114: 'The Lake Isle of Innisfree', in *The Rose* (1893) by W. B. Yeats, from *Collected Poems*, Vintage, 1992.

p.119: 'Burnt Norton', III, *Four Quartets*, by T. S. Eliot, Faber & Faber, 2001. Copyright © 1943 by T. S. Eliot. Reprinted with the permission of Faber & Faber.

p.120: 'Not Waving but Drowning' by Stevie Smith from *Collected Poems and Drawings of Stevie Smith*, Faber & Faber, 2015. Copyright © 1957 by Stevie Smith. Reprinted with the permission of Faber & Faber.

p.123: 'Nellie the Elephant', by Ralph Butler and Peter Hart, Parlophone, 1956.

p.158–159: *Alice's Adventures in Wonderland* by Lewis Carroll, 1865.

p.161: *Prince Caspian* by C. S. Lewis, HarperCollins Children's Books, 2009. Copyright © 1951 by C. S. Lewis Pte. Ltd.

p.172: *The Lion, the Witch, and the Wardrobe* by C. S. Lewis, HarperCollins Children's Books, 2009. Copyright © 1950 by C. S. Lewis Pte. Ltd.

p.196: *Anger* by Charles Lamb, unknown date.

p.199: *The Conduct of Life*, Ralph Waldo Emerson, 1860.

p.204: *Macbeth*, Act II, Scene II, William Shakespeare.

p.222: *The Yellow Birds*, Kevin Powers, Little, Brown, 2012. Copyright © Kevin Powers 2012.

p.230: 'Anthem', from the album *The Future* by Leonard Cohen, Columbia Records. Copyright © Sony Music Entertainment 1992.

p.252: "Hope' Is The Thing With Feathers', by Emily Dickinson, from *The Poems of Emily Dickinson*, edited by Ralph W. Franklin, Harvard University Press, 2005.

p.263: *The Journals of Sylvia Plath 1950–1962*, by Sylvia Plath, edited by Karen V. Kukil, Faber & Faber, 2014. Copyright © The Estate of Sylvia Plath 2000.

31901065325930